# THE
# FOUR-PACK
## REVOLUTION

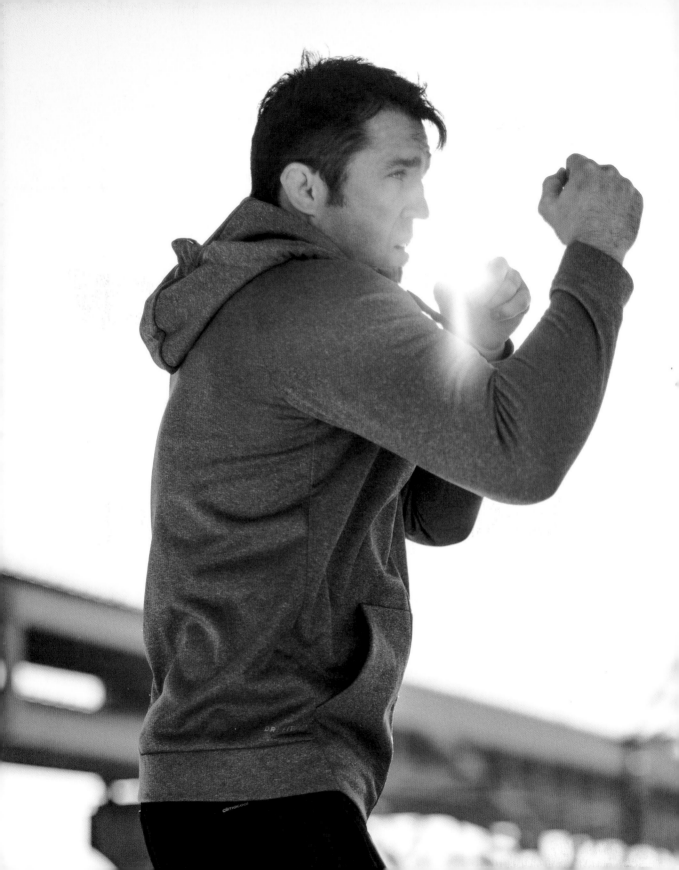

# THE FOUR-PACK REVOLUTION

## HOW YOU CAN AIM LOWER, CHEAT ON YOUR DIET, AND STILL LOSE WEIGHT AND KEEP IT OFF

# CHAEL SONNEN
### AND RYAN PARSONS

**RODALE.**

## RODALE
## *wellness*

*Live happy. Be healthy. Get inspired.*

Sign up today to get exclusive access to our authors, exclusive bonuses,
and the most authoritative, useful, and cutting-edge information on health, wellness,
fitness, and living your life to the fullest.

**Visit us online at RodaleWellness.com**
**Join us at RodaleWellness.com/Join**

© 2017 by Chael Sonnen and Ryan Parsons

All rights reserved. No part of this publication may be reproduced or transmitted in any form or by any means, electronic or mechanical, including photocopying, recording, or any other information storage and retrieval system, without the written permission of the publisher.

Rodale books may be purchased for business or promotional use for special sales.
For information, please e-mail: BookMarketing@Rodale.com.

Printed in the United States of America

Rodale Inc. makes every effort to use acid-free ♾, recycled paper ♻.

Photographs by Matthew Brush, except page 5 by Glenn Honiball, pages xii, 17, and 24 © Getty Images, page 40 courtesy of Casey Galpin, and page 89 courtesy of Ryan Parsons

Book design by Joanna Williams

Library of Congress Cataloging-in-Publication Data is on file with the publisher.

ISBN 978-1-62336-963-7 paperback

Distributed to the trade by Macmillan

2  4  6  8  10  9  7  5  3  1   paperback

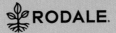

**RODALE**

We inspire health, healing, happiness, and love in the world.
Starting with you.

# CONTENTS

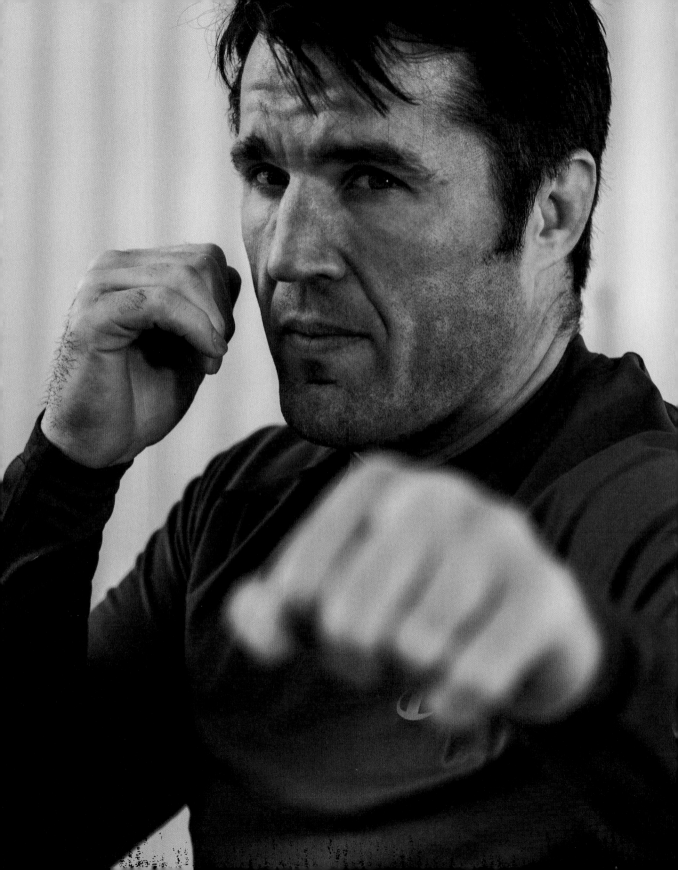

# CALL IT A COMEBACK

## MY JOURNEY BACK TO THE CAGE

**T**HERE WAS A LOT THAT NEEDED TO HAPPEN FOR MY COMEBACK TO MIXED martial arts to go from pipe dream to reality. I had been out of the fight game for over two years. That's two years away from serious training. Plus, I was two years older. Don't let anyone tell you age doesn't matter. It matters. You have to get smarter with each passing year or your body will not hold up.

The first real hurdle was passing a drug test. The reason for my two-year hiatus was that I had been flagged for using performance enhancing drugs (PEDs) 18 months earlier. When that hammer dropped, my life changed and it was time for a fresh start. When the day came to be retested, I was worried that there would be some residue left in my body. Since my suspension, the Ultimate Fighting Championship had implemented a new drug testing program run by the United States Anti-Doping Agency (USADA). This is the same agency that tests our nation's Olympic athletes. The UFC demonstrated its new commitment to the health and safety of its fighters by hiring Jeff Novitzky, the same guy who busted Lance Armstrong and Victor Conte's BALCO lab, to run its new drug testing program. After 20 years as a federal investigator, Novitzky had a reputation as someone who would do whatever it took to catch anyone breaking the rules. While the old drug testing procedures were widely considered to be a joke, the new program was now the strictest in any sport—amateur or professional. I had no margin for error and no more chances. It was 100 percent guaranteed that I would be tested the moment my name was entered into the testing pool. I imagined USADA would test both urine and blood with the latest scientific equipment, and save a portion of the sample for the future when even better testing procedures would be available. If I tested positive for anything, my mixed martial arts (MMA) career would be over. I'd probably have to start pro wrestling in Japan for $400 a week.

It turned out there was nothing to worry about. Despite extended testing, there was no evidence of PEDs or any other illegal substances in my system. Now I was faced with the task of rebuilding myself mentally and physically as I prepared to step back into the cage to compete in the toughest sport in the world. I also had to make sure the California State Athletic Commission would issue a license for me to fight as well as convince a promoter to give me a shot at redemption–and, hopefully, a huge paycheck. Despite the issues with the commission and not knowing if an organization would sign me, getting back in shape was what concerned me the most. During my break, I gained a substantial amount of weight. At my heaviest, I was 258 pounds–and it wasn't impressive. It was considerably more than the 185-pound weight class to which I hoped to return. So a year before my suspension was up, I started a 12-month clock in my head. If it was going to happen, it had to begin somewhere. Cue the music. I hope you're not imagining a Rocky Balboa–style training montage. If you are, prepare to be disappointed. Here's how this really went down.

When training for a fight, my primary workout is MMA training, which consists of 90 minutes of intense, technical drills, and live sparring and grappling. It's never easy. At 258 pounds, I thought to myself, "I can't do this." I knew how hard it was and how I was going to feel attempting it, so I avoided the gym altogether. At the time, this seemed like the best solution. In addition to sport-specific MMA training, I run a three-and-a-half-mile loop near my house for cardiovascular conditioning. But I was so heavy, I realized I couldn't complete that either. How did I know? When I walked up the stairs in my house, I'd be out of breath by the time I got to the top. That's how out of shape I was. Thankfully my trainer, Clayton, realized what was happening.

"All right, here's what you're going to do," he said. "Every time you go up stairs, I want you to do it as quickly as possible." He didn't make it about losing weight or even my comeback. It was never about fighting for a championship or setting a new personal record on my three-and-a-half-mile run. All I had to do was get up those stairs as quickly

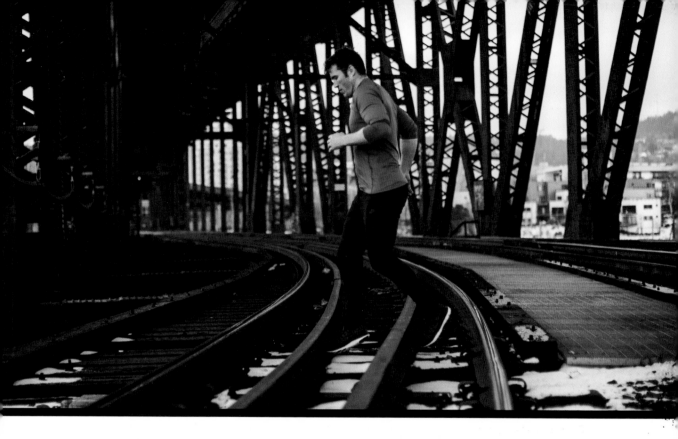

as possible—all 18 of them. This may seem insignificant on the surface, but every time I went up those stairs, I challenged myself to see how fast I could do it. This was the beginning of my return.

I also needed to change my diet, which was the driving force behind my weight gain. Starting small, my first step was eliminating soda. I was drinking four a day, which may not seem like a big deal, but replacing each can with water shaved 600 calories and 154 grams of sugar from my daily diet. It did not take long to see results. In the coming weeks, I added to my workouts and continued to refine my diet.

This was the process. There was no remote mountain training in the snow or fancy high-tech equipment monitoring my progress. I started one step at a time. It might not have been sexy, but this approach had teeth. Frequently the best solutions are simple, but simple isn't always easy. There were more obstacles to face, and I accepted each one of them and new challenges await me today. We all get to make a choice—adapt and overcome our problems or fall victim to them. I refuse to be a victim.

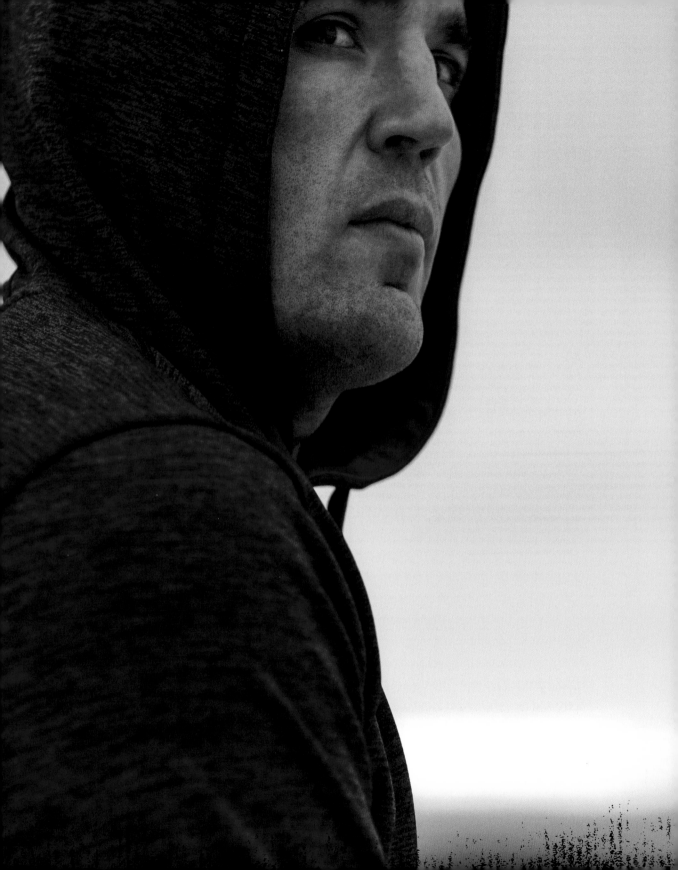

# INTRODUCTION

## LOWER YOUR EXPECTATIONS.
## PLAN FOR FAILURE.
## PREPARE FOR SUCCESS.

**YOU WAIT BEHIND THE CURTAIN LIKE KING KONG—THE MAIN ATTRACTION.**
Your pulse thumps like a drum, drowning out the cheers and muffled music. The months of sacrifice have left your body looking like it's been carved from granite. Your stomach churns with nervous energy and excitement—a thirst.

Not for victory or glory . . . but for water.

You've been dehydrating your body and restricting your caloric intake to make weight for this fight, and it worked. Now, on weigh-in day, you're in the best shape of your life. As you step out from behind the curtain you are greeted with an assault of flashbulbs, cheers, and raucous boos. Out of the corner of your eye, your opponent emerges. He is your date in the cage tomorrow night, an event that will be broadcast to millions around the world.

Stripping to your underwear, you feel yourself flex as thousands of Brazilian fans begin chanting, "*Uh vai morrer!*" This roughly translates to "YOU WILL DIE!" At least they don't mince words.

Months of training twice a day. A strict, finely tuned diet. It's taken a tremendous amount of mental and physical discipline to bring your body to this point. It's so difficult to maintain this body-fat percentage that it can only be achieved a few times a year—and it doesn't last long.

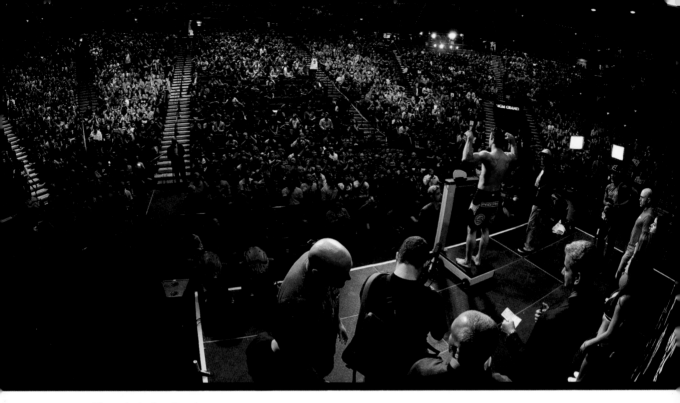

The calm before the storm

As the commission announces that you've made weight, relief floods your body, like it's been submerged in a warm bath. But quickly you're back at attention as your eyes find your opponent. You turn to face him and focus on your target. He's the reason you are here. You stand inches from each other's faces, your stares already grappling, locked in a hold. The crowd roars. You came for a fight—and tomorrow night, you're going to get one. Fists up. Pose for the cameras.

That image will be shared across hundreds of websites and thousands of Twitter feeds. The casual fan may think this is what fighters look like all year round—solidly defined, yoked-up machines—but that's not the case, and this scenario is not exclusive to fighters. The fitness model flexing on the cover of a magazine doesn't roll out of bed on any given day looking flawless, either. During the photo shoot, they are severely dehydrated and have starved themselves to achieve that desired "shredded" look. Not to mention, they are at the peak of their physical conditioning, as well as the beneficiaries of some pretty exceptional genes. And truth be told, many of them are also on steroids.

Steroids are not just prevalent in professional and amateur athletics anymore. Many in Hollywood and the fitness industry also rely on artificial means to achieve their incredible physiques. If the image still doesn't look quite right after the photo shoot, not to worry: The problem area will be fixed with the magic of Photoshop.

Looking like these fighters or cover models is the goal many of us strive for. But we have been defrauded by diet books and workout programs designed to trick us into believing we too can achieve a perfect physique. Perhaps, like the professionals, some of us could come close to this ideal state, but attempting to maintain this look for any reasonable amount of time while living a normal life is a recipe for disappointment and despair. Still, the allure of a six-pack is tempting. We want to believe anyone who promises to help us get one, and we will do some pretty silly things in the process.

Remember the electric pads that attached to your abs? The electric current making your muscles twitch was guaranteed to burn the fat off your belly, revealing a six-pack. Can you believe that product actually made it to market? It wasn't that long ago either. We're not sure how many people spent their hard-earned money on this modern-day snake oil, but it did sell. It's not hard to imagine someone sitting on the couch in front of their TV, abs twitching away, desperately hoping that this would be the solution to their problem. How many ab-zapping sessions did it take before the device ended up in the junk drawer with the old power cords and cables that no one knows what to do with? This is just one example of many fitness scams that have come and gone over the years that have promised to deliver a six-pack. None of them ever worked. And unfortunately, a few people got rich from someone else's misery. To anyone with a basic understanding of human physiology, these gimmicks have always seemed like foolish approaches to weight loss. (At least the Snuggie keeps you warm at night.)

The truth is, we would be the first in line to spend money on a pill or magic machine that delivered weight loss without effort. The concept of something for nothing is universally appealing—but that's not how life works. You have to do the work. You must give yourself time and, most importantly, remain consistent. There is no other way.

We have helped many athletes make weight for wrestling and mixed martial arts competitions, and by the time they step on the scale they are often sporting a good old-fashioned six-pack. But this is a side effect of intense physical preparation and sacrifice, not the goal. A highly refined, calorie reduced diet combined with dehydration and suffering led to that six-pack. Unfortunately, the level of discipline required to maintain that look is almost impossible to sustain for anyone living a normal life. Getting to this level of fitness is all these athletes do—it's their full-time job. Could you realistically live such a restricted life? Better question: do you want to? We'd like to have our cake and eat it too, but consider what happens to professional athletes when their careers are over—their peak physique disappears quickly. Even when fighters lose 30 pounds or more in the weeks leading up to a fight, it's a temporary state. The majority of them regain the weight within days after competition.

Here's what the fantasy weight-loss experience looks like for most of us.

- **Day 1:** Your morning starts with a green shake and 27 minutes on the elliptical. When you pop on the scale at midday you are delighted to discover you've already lost 4 pounds! Momentum and euphoria carry you through the day.
- **Day 3:** Your cravings are gone. With more energy, you move with a bounce in your step and you haven't slept better in years. Total weight loss to date: 8 pounds.
- **Day 7:** You hit your target weight. Shopping for new clothes is fun, your abs are back, all 8 of them, and people notice the changes. Time to celebrate.
- **Day 14:** You go to the beach with friends in your new Jeep. Everyone gasps as you take your shirt off. You flex your abs and smile. Good things happen to good people.

But you probably identify more with the following:

- **Day 1:** After months of procrastination, you finally decide to join a gym. Throughout the first workout, your body and mind rebel with every repetition.
- **Day 3:** Unbelievably, despite 7 hours of exercise and four weight-loss shakes over the past 3 days, you've managed to gain a pound. You are sore. Waves of pain hit your muscles with every breath. At 10:30 p.m. you stare into your fridge, hoping a plate of orange chicken will magically appear. You reluctantly scarf down some organic blueberries and go to sleep.
- **Day 7:** You've lost 2 pounds, your mood fluctuates with the wind, and although no one has told you, you're not that fun to be around. The soreness is beginning to fade, but your cravings seem to escalate.

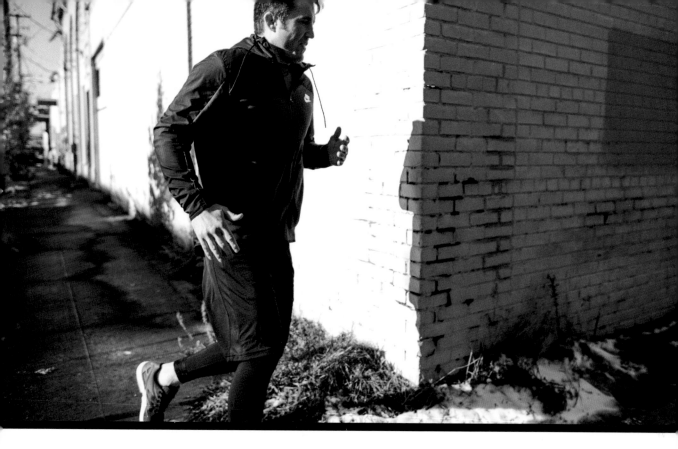

- **Day 10:** You go out for drinks with friends, eat tacos at 3:00 a.m., and sleep off the booze the following day. Nothing quells a hangover quite like greasy food. Taking the weekend off from the gym, you say to yourself, "I'll start again on Monday."
- **Day 28:** You have repeated this cycle twice. Weight loss to date: half a pound.

The sad and unfortunate part of this scenario is that you were doomed to fail. Unrealistic expectations and a misguided approach have left millions of people feeling helpless, frustrated, and defeated. We're offering a different approach. Lower your standards. Plan for failure. Prepare for success. By doing so, a strong, healthy mind and body are within reach.

So stop pursuing an unattainable six-pack. Instead, aim for a four-pack, where the top two-thirds of your abs are showing. A four-pack is achievable while still enjoying life. It's the wave of the future.

Here's why. Genetics play a major role in what can be achieved, especially when it concerns your physique. Unfortunately, most of us naturally have a hard time losing the fat that covers the lower portion of our abs. Because of this, a six-pack is extremely difficult for most people to obtain, especially for anyone over the age of 17. Even those of us who can achieve a six-pack often find it virtually impossible to sustain.

For the record, there are people who are naturally lean and tend to be blessed with small appetites and fast metabolisms. For them, gaining weight is the challenge. Don't compare yourself. They were dealt a different set of cards, and we can only play the hand we hold. A four-pack is realistic for most of us. Not only will you look good, you'll feel good, which is something we can't say for those hungry six-pack people. This frees you to enjoy other activities besides obsessing about your diet and body-fat percentage. Your friends and family will be ever so grateful.

We are all unique, and each of our bodies responds differently to diet and exercise. Some of us seem to gain 6 pounds after eating a plate of pasta, while others are less sensitive to carbohydrates. Your body today may have a different response to foods than it did 20 years ago. You are constantly evolving and changing, even if at first glance life feels stagnant. Healthy living is not a static state. Balancing proper eating habits and workout regimens with the stress of daily life requires consistent but doable maintenance.

Setting your sights on a four-pack is an achievable, realistic, and sustainable goal. Our mission is to assist you in breaking the cycle of failure and bad habits that have kept you from making lasting progress. Since there are multiple ways to create a four-pack, our emphasis is on giving you the tools to discover what works best for you. That said, there is a basic set of principles that apply to everyone. After learning the fundamentals, your challenge will be to integrate these principles into your daily life.

A significant aspect of your four-pack strategy is learning how to deal with the bad days that will inevitably occur. If you are the type of person who believes you should not have any problems or if you avoid discomfort at all costs, you need to rethink your approach. In the wise words of Tony Robbins, "Your real problem may be that you think you shouldn't have any." There is no way to achieve your goals by staying in your comfort zone. Your best self is forged from sacrifice. The mindset to rely on when times get tough is perfectly defined by the Finnish word *sisu*, which means "continuing to act in the face of repeated failures and extreme odds." Throughout your four-pack journey, you can rely on a sisu mindset to overcome any obstacle.

# FIRST MOVES

1. **TAKE A SHIRTLESS PICTURE.** You don't have to share it with anyone, it's just for you. As you lose weight, refer to this picture as a reminder of how far you've come. Elite athletes rely on coaches to maintain perspective, and the Four-Pack Revolution will do the same for you.

2. **ANNOUNCE YOUR PLAN TO FRIENDS.** This isn't about trying to impress them. It's about accountability. Some may roll their eyes, others may support you, and a few may actually join in. Plus, no one wants to look like a failure. Anything you can do to create leverage for yourself is helpful.

You may initially skip over these steps—that's okay. But consider coming back to them as you read further and strengthen your four-pack commitment. These small steps may be where you need to begin. But before we get into the specifics of the Four-Pack Revolution program, let's take a look at the current health and fitness landscape and see what you're up against.

The most damaging mistake many people make when attempting to lose weight is allowing one misstep to throw them off course. Before they know it, 6 months pass and the scale reads 15 pounds heavier. If you slip and drink a few beers and eat a burger, that's fine—make up for it with your next meal. No matter where you are or what mistakes you've made, there's always a route back. And often the distance is much shorter than you have anticipated. A few simple tweaks can change the direction of your life. Don't burn the house down when things don't go your way. Stay the course. Adapt. *Sisu*.

It's helpful to learn from others because we often make the same few mistakes: starting too fast, setting unrealistic expectations, and not having a plan B for when plan A stops yielding results. So before that happens, here are some tips that will help you establish the right mindset for this journey.

- **Don't seek comfort:** Aim for fulfillment, which will support you on days when you're feeling frustrated. Comfort is easy to come by but rarely produces significant results. It's often paired with excuses and blame in order to lessen the pain of not living up to your expectations. Leave those thoughts behind and remember that fulfillment leads to an extraordinary life. Embrace the challenge, take a deep breath, and step up. Learn to manage your discomfort and discover joy in the work. The biggest battle is the one fought between your ears, so win the mental game and the rest will be easy.

- **Adjust your point of view:** You know exactly why you are out of shape. Knowing how to change is where everyone gets stuck because there is more involved than just diet and exercise. You need to invest time in altering how you view your situation. If you don't believe change is possible, you'll never mobilize the resources necessary to create lasting results. If you have attempted to make changes in the past and failed, remember that your own life is filled with examples where you have solved problems and found your way through tough situations. You've done it before and will do it again.

- **Expect to fail:** In most areas of life, it's not a good idea to expect failure. But when it comes to your diet, consider this: you are going to be eating several times a day, every day, for the rest of your life. So factor in a margin for error. Do you know what they call a baseball player who fails almost 70 percent of the time? An all-star. Don't waste time wallowing in failure–refocus and get ready to go.

- **Lower your expectations:** "But wait," you say. "I would never lower my expectations. I want the best of everything." Most people set unrealistic goals about what's possible in the near term, which leads to frustration and an increased risk of failure. This is not the ideal foundation for any weight-loss plan. You can always raise the bar as you go. Set obtainable goals and celebrate small victories. It's a long road, so don't be afraid to stop and admire the progress you've made. Imagine what you can accomplish with 12 months of focused effort. Your life can and will be significantly different.

Ready to get started? In the coming chapters, we'll lay out all the tools needed to create a new and enhanced version of yourself that will cut a great shape in a suit and look good poolside in Vegas.

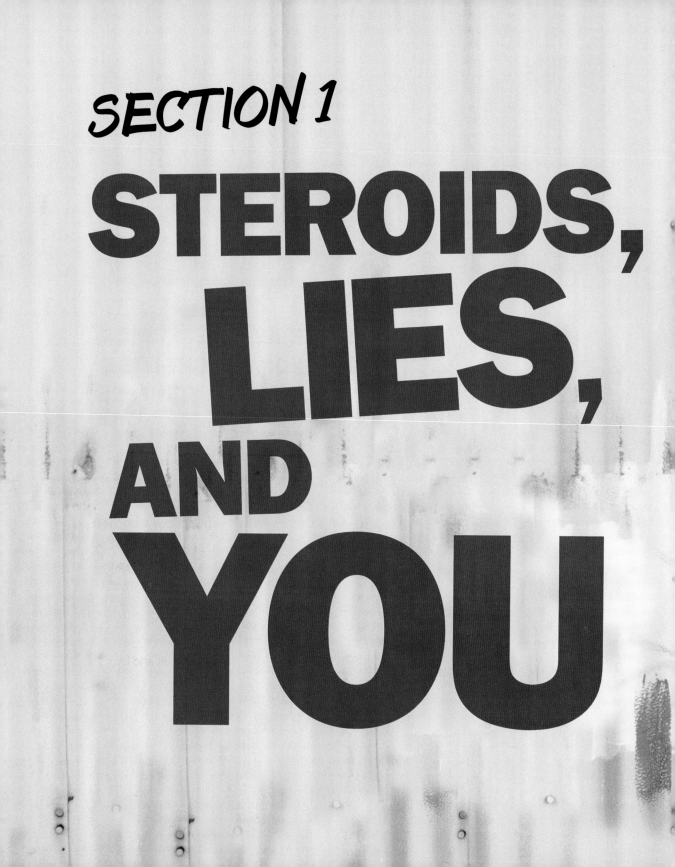

SECTION 1

# STEROIDS, LIES, AND YOU

# 1
# LOOK AROUND

## THE TRUTH ABOUT STEROIDS, PHOTOSHOP, WEIGHT-LOSS BOOKS, AND MMA FIGHTERS

**Y**EARS AGO, RETURNING FROM AN ULTIMATE FIGHTING CHAMPIONSHIP EVENT in Columbus, Ohio, where the Arnold Classic was taking place, we chatted with a professional female fitness competitor at the airport. Fitness competitors are not overblown cartoon characters like bodybuilders have become. They are in amazing condition, but they're much smaller and don't look like freak shows. Although our new friend had just finished competing, her carry-on luggage consisted entirely of meals for the trip home, with each portion of food carefully weighed out in plastic containers. She was happy to talk with us about her lifestyle as a professional fitness competitor, and readily admitted that every one of her opponents regularly injects a cocktail consisting of several different types of performance enhancing drugs. Every. Single. One.

Steroids are rampant in professional sports, not just in fitness competitions and bodybuilding. Each athlete falls into one of three categories: those who use, those who don't use, and those who lie about it. This is not groundbreaking news. Ask any (honest) professional football player and they'll tell you. Everyone is battling to cash in on that one big contract, but the shelf life of an NFL player is incredibly short. In a league with the least amount of guaranteed money and the largest amount of long-term damaging effects, athletes will do almost anything to get paid before it's too late. On top of that, it is hard to recover by Monday morning from repeated high-speed collisions with 300-pound linemen the afternoon before. When everyone else is using performance enhancing drugs, there's enormous pressure to do the same just to keep the playing field even.

Mixed martial arts is no exception. You don't need to look far to find a number of high-profile athletes who have tested positive. Until recently, the sport had very lax drug testing policies and the majority of fighters who used never got caught. Now that the UFC has implemented Olympic-level testing, there have been dramatic changes in the physiques of athletes on fight night. It's even ended some careers. There have been fighters who have opted to retire rather than compete naturally, and even more who were suddenly not as invincible as they were in the pre-USADA drug testing days.

The team at USADA is very successful at catching athletes who cheat. If someone is using, chances are they will eventually get caught. With each technical improvement in the precisely calibrated equipment used to detect steroids, more athletes' secrets are exposed. Since the International Olympic Committee started retesting old samples from previous Olympics with advanced technology, at least six athletes from the 2008 and 2012 Games have been stripped of their medals and hundreds of positive tests for heavy-duty anabolic steroids have been revealed.

In 2014, the *Washington Post* reported on a German documentary in which former Russian discus thrower Yevgeniya Pecherina claimed that "99 percent of athletes selected to represent Russia in international competition use banned substances." The same article states the Russian Athletics Federation (RAF) and the International Association of Athletics Federations (IAAF) hid positive tests. There are rumors that this cover-up goes all the way to the Russian president, Vladimir Putin. The Russian track and field team was not allowed to compete at the 2016 Olympic Games in Rio de Janeiro. Imagine what it would take for a country as large and powerful as Russia to have so many athletes banned. There was a lot of abuse.

## HAVE YOU EVER REALLY LOOKED AT THE FITNESS MODEL ON THE MAGAZINE COVER?

There's a dirty little secret no one likes to talk about–most fitness models are not natural. While you were stuck at the office working overtime, that genetically gifted specimen in his physical prime was training twice a day. It's his full-time job. In the weeks leading up to the photo shoot, he dramatically cut his calories to an unhealthy level, and was almost completely dehydrated at the moment the photo was taken. To add to the mix, he's likely been taking performance enhancing drugs (PEDs). Yes, that's right–he's taking steroids, too. PEDs have become so prevalent that many people have started to believe it's normal to look like these athletes and models. With so many diet and supplement companies promoting this look–promising to "flush" fat out and help you achieve a Superman six-pack physique–you would think it's achievable for anyone. Sadly, this marketing strategy puts entirely unrealistic expectations on the rest of us.

But the fitness industry's conspiracy against you isn't always as dramatic as steroid abuse. Spend 30 seconds on YouTube and you'll witness the transformative power a Photoshop artist wields. Magazine photos were getting this treatment long before the digital age, so it's unlikely you have ever seen an advertising image that has not been retouched—from weight-loss before-and-afters to automobile ads. Not to mention the wonders makeup and lighting do before an image even makes it into the photo editor's hands. You see these doctored photos on product labels, book covers, magazine articles, and advertisements. The saturation of this "look" into our minds is total. If this is the standard we hold ourselves to for beauty and fitness, what hope does the average person have? None—these fictionalized images have set you up to fail.

Let's not forget about those UFC weigh-ins. I fought a good portion of my career in the UFC at 185 pounds. Now, it would be reasonable to think I actually weighed 185 pounds, but that's far from the truth. Combat-sports athletes have cut weight for as long as there have been weight classes in an attempt to gain a competitive advantage. In a fist-fight, it's usually better to be bigger and stronger than your opponent. The truth is, apart from the few weeks leading up to a fight, I usually weighed over 220 pounds. Losing 35 pounds in a short period of time is dangerous and filled with suffering, but it's part of a fighter's job. If you're wondering how I did it, the first half of the weight comes off by following the diet advice dished out in this book. The balance of the weight loss is accomplished by torture in a hot sauna and dramatically reducing food and water intake to potentially lethal levels. Exactly what you do not want to do. These are the sacrifices amateur wrestlers and professional MMA fighters make, but there is a price to pay. You can

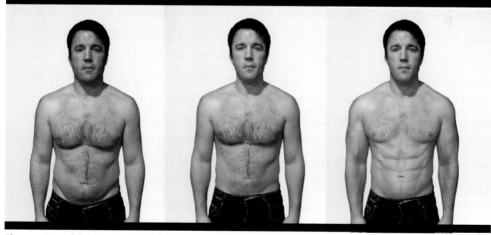

*Three versions of the same image—only two have been retouched*

only do this so many times before your body starts fighting back. There have been a number of confirmed deaths as a result of weight cutting. In the first six weeks of the 1997 NCAA wrestling season, three college wrestlers died cutting weight. Their tragic deaths sparked the NCAA to make changes to reduce the incidence of severe weight cutting. Unfortunately, these young men were not the last to pay the ultimate price. Just a few months ago, a Scottish muay Thai fighter died wearing a plastic sweat suit in an attempt to cut weight for an upcoming bout.

What athletes and models go through to achieve a certain weight can almost be described as a situational eating disorder. Often they develop a complete obsession with their diet and weight loss. Diuretics, laxatives, starvation, and occasionally bulimia are some of the extreme methods used. As you read on, you will realize why this approach is so detrimental. So don't be too impressed with the physique of a severely dehydrated, malnourished professional fighter or fitness model—you should have much higher standards for your life.

## THE SIX-PACK SEDUCTION

Everyone wants one, but in real life, six-packs are mostly found on the young, the juiced, or the genetically blessed. You know, those guys who can smash seven slices of meat lover's pizza and wake up with an extra ab. Screw them—they're not reading this book anyway. It's very difficult to make life changes knowing that the odds are overwhelmingly against you. You may not admit that consciously, but there's a part of you that knows your expectations may not be entirely realistic. At minute 32 on the Stairmaster, it's easy to imagine yourself shirtless and ripped, dunking a basketball at the park. That may work fine as motivation to get you through one cardio session, but ultimately that image can be destructive, sabotaging your success. Instead, consider lowering your expectations.

A four-pack, on the other hand, is achievable for most us. Whether you're a full-time student, a parent, a workaholic, or the guy who loves lounging around on the couch, you can achieve a four-pack while still enjoying life. Why a four-pack? First of all, it is impossible to reduce body fat in one specific area. That concept is called "spot reduction" and, despite decades of fitness products promising to melt away stubborn belly fat, the human body does not work that way. When you start to lose weight and your body-fat percentage decreases, the fat that covers your lower abs is usually the last to go. That's just how it is. But with a few simple adjustments to your diet and lifestyle, your upper and middle abs can be revealed, giving you a healthy, sustainable four-pack. You'll look great in clothes and can feel good taking your shirt off at the beach, all while protecting yourself from the preventable, deadly diseases that plague modern society like diabetes, heart disease, and stroke. Sure, you won't look like a magazine cover model—but no one will call you fat. And seeing four of your six abs when you flex in the mirror is quite satisfying.

## ARE YOU PALEO, BRO?

It's difficult keeping up with the latest diet and fitness industry trends. For years we have been inundated with captivating diets that have swept through pop culture. Since numerous diet gurus all have something to say about losing weight, let's clear the air. The truth is that you can find short-term success with almost any diet. But are they good for you? Low-fat diets were popular for years, but they led to unnecessary suffering, as have high-protein diets that forbid carbohydrates. While history has shown us that it's possible to lose weight by following a variety of programs, the vast majority of dieters can't keep it off. When you restrict food intake significantly or eat foods that you don't enjoy, you're more prone to breaking down, bingeing, and disrupting your metabolism.

Trendy diets may help you hit your 30-day goal, but 6 months down the line you'll most likely be sitting at plus-10 pounds from where you started. Even when positive changes are made, limited focus and energy are spent acquiring the new habits needed to sustain weight loss. Because of these fad diets and their touted "successes," many of us end up riding a manic diet swing, drastically changing our diets and workouts to lose weight as quickly as possible on one end, and eating like we just don't give a damn on the other. There is a better way.

## YOU ARE WHO YOU ARE

Pay close attention, as this piece of advice will save you years of pain and frustration: Quit comparing your body to someone else's. (For the women reading: Yes, guys do this, too.) If you are 5-foot-8 with a naturally stocky build, you can never look like a 6-foot-2 model, for the same reason Kim Kardashian will never look like Kate Moss. There are pros and cons to any body type. Some people are built to move fast; others do better at a slow, steady pace. You are who you are.

Great coaches and general managers select athletes based on body type all the time. The most obvious example is in gymnastics, a sport that requires a very specific build that people are either born with or not. A coach with a trained eye knows exactly which child from a very early age has the potential to develop into a competitive gymnast. Think about the way football prospects are scouted. Every inch of them is measured. Each position on the field has its own prototypical or ideal size. In other sports, such as wrestling and mixed martial arts (MMA), there are a variety of body types that can be successful. For you MMA fans, it's obvious that Mark Hunt can't look or move like Dominick Cruz. Both are incredible fighters, but physically they could not be more different. Each athlete must develop a style that suits his or her genetic makeup. Some are slow and grind their way to victory, while others are explosive and rely on athleticism to get the job done.

Professional models face similar hurdles. You were either born with the potential to be a supermodel or not. Does the distance between your eyes and the shape of your nose fit certain cultural standards that are considered attractive? Does the ratio of your leg length to your torso give you a look designers think will best show off their clothes? No matter how hard a voluptuous 5-foot-2 woman tries to look like a classic runway model, it is not going to happen.

While good genetic makeup is no guarantee of success, it does provide an advantage. That said, no matter what your genetic predisposition, there's a healthy, in-shape version of yourself that looks great if given the opportunity. Despite our unique differences, there are basic foundations for a healthy diet and exercise regime that apply to all of us. By recognizing and accepting who you are instead of trying to emulate someone else, you'll have a better chance of success. Your job will be to take the information in this book and make it work in your life. Only you can make it happen.

To get started, take a moment to judge the distance between where you are now and where you'd like to be. This "gap" helps determine how long you should expect the process to take. Be specific about what you're attempting to accomplish; "I want to lose weight" isn't enough. This reflection is important for three reasons.

1. Targeted goals create long-term vision for your life. If you know where you want to be, it becomes easier to measure your progress.

2. Refined effort, not aimless hard work, is what's required—and this is where so many people fail. Having systems in place and a plan for your day ensures your actions create impact.

3. Lastly, it's easier to remain consistent if your goals are congruent with your interests and values. The way you approach food and exercise must fit with your personality. Not everyone is the 5:00 a.m. yoga class type.

How long will it take? As we have previously said, everyone's a little different, but the following chart gives you an estimate of what to expect.

- <10 pounds: 4–8 weeks
- 10–20 pounds: 8–20 weeks
- 21–30 pounds: 3–7 months
- 31–40 pounds: 5–10 months
- 41–50 pounds: 8–14 months

If you are significantly overweight, your initial weight loss may occur at a rapid pace. If you lose 5 or more pounds in the first week, most of that will come from retained water. Losing this water weight is still a positive step forward—as long you don't expect to maintain this pace. Be aware that your progress will slow down and when it does, managing expectations will be just as important as what you eat.

## SURVEY THE LANDSCAPE

We have made remarkable strides as a society in the past 30 years with advances in technology, medicine, and communication. The fitness and health food industries have evolved as well. There are endless free online workouts and more organic juice bars than ever before, and things seem to be looking up—but it's all window dressing. The fact is the average American weighs 25 pounds more than he or she did 30 years ago. As we grow as a nation, so does our collective waistline. This is not just a problem in the United States, though. The situation is also dire abroad. Between 1958 and 1962, 36 million people starved to death during the Great Famine in China; today, Chinese kids are almost as overweight as Americans are. As countries develop, obesity rates tend to rise in concert with their GDP. Japan is the world's only wealthy country with an obesity rate below 10 percent. If you've ever been to Japan, you know just how different a "large" T-shirt is compared to one sold at Walmart. Their version of a large looks like it would fit the average American fifth-grader. This isn't surprising when you consider that the size of a stack of pancakes at the Japanese version of a restaurant like Denny's is half the size of its counterpart in the US. Same goes for soft drinks—good luck finding a Big Gulp at a Japanese convenience store. With all the steps forward we've taken as a modern society, our health has backpedaled.

In some ways, despite more dietary resources being available, it's easier than ever to let our weight spiral out of control. While fruits and vegetables have increased in price by up to 91 percent over the past 25 years, the cost of processed foods, high in sugar and unhealthy fats, has become considerably less expensive. If you blame your budget on not being able to eat healthy food, consider this: while you can get a burger, fries, and soda for six bucks at a fast food joint, a healthy, home-cooked dinner can be made for half that.

Combined with the rise of digital entertainment and decreased physical activity, it's clear to see how this obesity epidemic has spun out of control. It's never been easier to be entertained and connected while sitting still. Going outside to play is a foreign concept to many kids, and most teenagers would prefer a phone to a car. There is less incentive to move when the world is at your fingertips. We are living in different times, and these two forces—processed food and modern technology—have dramatically altered our society. From how children are raised to the way people work, many aspects of our lives are dramatically different from a generation ago, for good and bad. Taking a look at how you have adapted your life to these social changes can highlight specific areas for improvement.

It's tough to fight modern science. Ryan once consulted for an international company that was launching an energy drink. Scientists from a prominent food development company were asked to create a beverage that customers would want to frequently consume. Spending time in a modern food-science lab was eye-opening. The taste, color, mouth-feel, and addictive qualities were all manipulated so the customer would keep coming back for more. Think of what happens when a tube of Pringles is opened. From our experience, those chips have a pretty short lifespan (let's not even discuss how long a package of Thin Mints might last). They were engineered by highly trained food scientists to target your cravings.

What's even more alarming is that the tastes you grew up with tend to dominate your food choices as an adult. So if you were raised in the South with a steady diet of fried chicken and mac and cheese, odds are you will carry those preferences throughout your life.

It's understandable, then, why losing weight can be such a challenge, because we are fighting a two-front war against genetics and technology. If you are raising kids or plan to at some point, this is something to consider. They will only know what you expose them to in those early years.

So, let's review the facts. The National Health and Nutrition Examination Survey completed in 2009–2010 gave us these scary statistics.

- More than 2 in 3 American adults are considered to be overweight.

- More than 1 in 3 American adults are considered to be obese.

- More than 1 in 20 American adults are considered to be extremely obese.

- About 1 in 3 of American children and adolescents ages 6 to 19 are considered to be overweight or obese.

- More than 1 in 6 American children and adolescents ages 6 to 19 are considered to be obese.

Translation: Without considerable effort to reverse this trend, the health of our society is doomed. It will require the combined efforts of businesses, government, schools, religious institutions, and families to solve the problem. On the bright side, there is nothing preventing you from stopping your contribution to this cycle and reversing course. This involves rethinking your relationship with food. Consider how college students consume alcohol at a fraternity party; it is very different from a couple's night out when you're 35. Remember Halloween when you were 8 years old and made yourself sick from eating so much candy? Hopefully you do things a little differently now.

# 10 LIES YOU'VE BEEN TOLD ABOUT WEIGHT LOSS

The sheer volume of misinformation regarding weight loss makes this subject difficult to navigate. While the basic principles of losing weight are simple, experts often make the process more difficult than it needs to be. So let's address the top 10 weight-loss myths before moving forward.

## LIE #1:
### A Calorie Is a Calorie

Your body metabolizes various foods in different ways. Proteins, fats, and carbohydrates have diverse effects on your hunger, blood sugar, and hormonal responses. One calorie of protein is not the same as a calorie of sugar. For example, 250 calories from a grilled chicken breast can boost your metabolism and reduce appetite and cravings, but 250 calories from a can of soda will spike your blood sugar and may affect your mood and energy level. Calories from whole, natural sources are generally more filling than refined, processed foods.

## LIE #2:
### Losing Weight Is a Linear Process

Your weight can fluctuate daily by several pounds depending on when you weigh yourself, how much water you're retaining, and the type of food you have recently eaten. Tracking healthy, long-term weight loss will show an overall downward trend with periods of small gains and occasional plateaus. So don't be surprised if it takes a few days for the scale to acknowledge your effort.

## LIE #3:
### Supplements Can Help You Lose Weight

Weight-loss pills are generally ineffective and a waste of your money. When the infomercial says you can lose weight without changing your diet–yes, it's too good to be true. Don't fall for it.

## LIE #4:
### Weight Loss Is about Willpower, Not Biology

Your ability to gain or lose weight is influenced by lifestyle and genetics. Relying on will-power alone is a losing battle. The only way to sustain change is to work with your body in a way that fits your personality and natural tendencies.

## LIE #5:
### You Should Eat Less and Exercise More

At first glance, this sounds entirely reasonable and true. And it probably is. But this advice is shortsighted and neglects a host of other factors that contribute to gaining weight. If you eat to relieve stress or have never exercised regularly, this requires a change in your habits and lifestyle. You'll need to find new ways to meet those emotional needs that will contribute to a healthier lifestyle. It's like advising someone who is broke to "just earn more money" or telling someone who is depressed to "be happy" or "snap out of it." If it were that easy, we would all be fit.

## LIE #6:
### Carbs Make You Fat

Humans have been eating carbohydrates for a long time. Reducing carbs—especially sugar—will help you lose weight, but you still need healthy carbohydrates in your diet, pri-marily from non-starchy veggies and legumes (beans). Think: less bread and pasta, more beans and water-rich vegetables.

## LIE #7:
### Fat Is Bad

Fat has gotten a bad rap for decades. In truth, as long as you don't overeat, fat will not make you fat. This essential nutrient makes food taste better and is needed by your body to function effectively. But just as there are good and bad carbs, there are also good and bad fats. Half an avocado is vastly different from an equal portion of refined vegetable oil.

# LIE #8:
## Eating Breakfast Is Necessary to Lose Weight

Chances are you're hungry when you wake up. It's been close to 10 hours since your last meal, so go eat! A small amount of protein in the morning will help carry you through the day. If you are one of those people without much of an appetite when you get up, it's not that big of a deal, but be prepared to eat something healthy later on. Stopping for a bagel or snacking at your desk won't cut it.

# LIE #9:
## Dieting Is Effective

Let's unpack this myth for a moment. Changing how you eat is obviously paramount to transforming your body. But "dieting," i.e., restricting yourself to one specific way of eating, is what we're attacking here. You will more than likely lose weight if you adhere to any diet, but the problem is maintaining that lifestyle. Eight-five percent of people who diet regain all the weight they lost within 12 months. So dieting is effective–for a time. But if you want your new physique to last longer than a weekend in Myrtle Beach, you'd better read on.

# LIE #10:
## "Diet" Foods Are Good for You

Learn to read nutritional labels, not big, bold marketing buzzwords on the front of a package. Foods with a high percentage of unnatural ingredients are best avoided. You may be surprised to discover how much sugar, additives, and unhealthy oils are contained in the diet foods and drinks you regularly consume, some of which may be labeled as natural or organic.

In the next few chapters, we will take a look at how many of our expectations about weight loss are unrealistic. We'll explore key influencers available now to help you lose weight and will help identify what's been holding you back. Whoever said, "If you find yourself in a hole, the first thing you should do is stop digging" was correct. It's not difficult to make a few simple changes that shift the momentum in your favor.

# 2
# LOOK INSIDE

## BEIJING, CHINA, AUGUST 19, 2008

Daniel Cormier was at the top of his game. Four weeks earlier, he made his second Olympic wrestling team, was named team captain of the US squad, and was among a small group of American athletes favored to bring home gold. Years of hard work, combined with exceptional talent, led him to reach a level few ever achieve.

Most wrestlers, especially at the elite level, choose to cut weight in order to compete at a lower weight class. Weight cutting was nothing new to Cormier. He had been competing his entire life and first started cutting weight at age 13 but, not surprisingly, he went about it the wrong way. A week before he had to weigh in, Daniel would wear a plastic sweat suit, dehydrating himself and placing tremendous stress on his body. In college he wrestled at 185 pounds—and never once missed weight. But what happens to most of us also happened to Cormier: As he got older, it became easier to pack on the pounds. This meant he had more weight to lose for each competition.

With less than a week before his weigh-in in Beijing, Cormier needed to lose 27 pounds to reach the limit of his weight class—211.5 pounds. The weight cut wasn't going well but this was the Olympic Games, and somehow Cormier found a way to lose the weight. Then the unthinkable happened.

In the hours after stepping off the scale, Cormier was rushed to a local Chinese hospital as his kidneys began shutting down. Even for an elite athlete in his prime, the stress of the weight cut on his body was too much. Despite the administration of intravenous fluids to replace the water and electrolytes he lost making weight, his health continued to deteriorate. His doctors knew he was in no shape to compete the next day and had no choice but to recommend that Cormier be pulled from Olympic competition before he ever had a chance to step on the mat. His Olympic dream was over. While Cormier lay in a hospital bed in Beijing, his would-be opponent walked onto the mat and, with the Olympic rings hanging overhead, had his hand raised in victory without ever breaking a sweat.

The pain of not being able to compete in the Olympic Games after years of sacrifice was difficult for Cormier to put into words. "I missed out on an opportunity to win an Olympic gold medal by not being disciplined and committed," Cormier told Fox Sports.

No one is immune to the side effects of bad choices, and at some point they catch up to you. But pain can be a great motivator, and Cormier was not the type to sit back and let this experience define who he was. His story was not over, and soon after the Olympics passed he changed his focus and began a career in mixed martial arts. Since his weight had ballooned to 264 pounds, he decided to compete as a heavyweight. He was clearly over his natural body weight, but his speed and athleticism were beneficial against larger opponents.

In 2014, after his second fight in the Ultimate Fighting Championship as a heavyweight, Cormier announced his intention to drop to light heavyweight–205 pounds, or

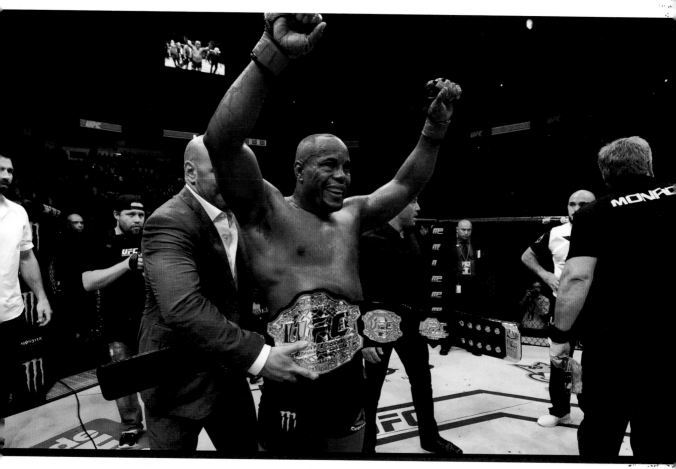

Seven years after a disastrous weight cup at the Olympic Games, Daniel Cormier becomes the UFC Light Heavyweight Champion.

6.5 pounds less than the weight he had trouble attaining for the Olympics years prior. Cormier possessed the technical, mental, and competitive skills to match up against anyone in the world, but this time his opponent was himself.

To make weight, Cormier had to change his eating habits. Growing up in the South gave him a love of unhealthy foods, and Popeyes chicken held a special place in his heart. At family meals, the only food left on the table at the end was the plate of vegetables. This is how his family ate when he was growing up. Cormier knew that for his life to change, he had to change—which is exactly what he did. Out went the Dr Pepper and fried chicken; in came veggies, slow-digesting carbs, and lean protein. And water. Lots of water.

This time around, things were different. Not only did Cormier make weight at 205 pounds, but 12 months later he was crowned UFC light heavyweight champion. All the pain stemming from mistakes in his past was erased, and his name as a champion was forever etched into the record books.

## LOOK WITHIN

While Cormier's diet caused him to miss competing in the Olympic Games, he had been eating unhealthily since childhood. We all tend to gravitate to what's comfortable. When faced with the prospect of uncertainty, it's easier to settle into familiar patterns than forge a new path. Cormier found a way around this, but not everyone does. This process involves understanding your psychology—the way you approach life—and your physiology: how your body responds to food, exercise, and stress.

Cormier had a difficult set of decisions to make if he was going to achieve his lifelong dream of becoming a world champion. Changing his approach to food was not an easy task, but the sacrifice was worth it. He will tell you that nothing ever tasted as good as the feeling of a 12-pound UFC championship belt around his waist. For Daniel, you, and the rest of us, creating lasting change hinges on our ability to separate our emotions from our decision-making process. This is a skill that can be developed with practice, so get started by asking yourself these three questions. Write your answers down and put them in a place where you can refer to them regularly.

1. **What do I really want?**

   There's a difference between what we think we want and what we really want. When these visions for our life are not aligned, lasting change becomes difficult to accomplish. The satisfaction of achieving goals is short-lived. When the applause and congratulations die down, an anxious feeling arises: Now what? In this moment, many people get lost, but knowing what drives you makes managing these times much easier.

2. **What has prevented me from succeeding in the past?**

   For most of us, the answer to this question stares back at us in the mirror each morning. If you could just get out of your own way, life would be so much easier. Take a moment to step back and examine how you typically respond to stress. What patterns or habits do you need to eliminate? Are there specific people, places, or situations that keep you from your best? What distractions do you use to avoid taking action?

3. **What three steps can I take right now to improve my situation?**

   Awareness is great, but unless it's paired with immediate action it doesn't mean a whole lot. Identifying simple next steps helps build momentum and confidence, and strengthens your ability to change.

We'll get into creating a winning mindset in Chapter 7 and how to build positive habits in Chapter 8, and give you all the tools you need to stay on track in Chapter 10. But first let's create a better understanding of your physiology and the key factors within your body that influence weight loss.

## INFLUENCERS

Your ability to lose weight isn't dependent on any single element. There are several factors that influence the process; your brain, metabolism, hormones, sleep, exercise, diet, and genetics are all leading contributors. Having a general understanding of the big picture and the role each influencer plays makes it easier to navigate the process while making better decisions.

## Your Brain

Your brain is a source of tremendous power, but it can also be your toughest adversary. If you're like most of us, you were never taught to control and direct your mind during childhood. As a result, you've most likely developed a few bad habits. Your brain craves instant gratification. Why wait for something when you can feel good now? Resorting to a "feel good now" mindset is a daily occurrence for many, and it's difficult to overcome with willpower alone. Learning to regulate impulse control is the first step toward harnessing the power of your brain to create change.

Impulse control is different than willpower, because it uses awareness and mindfulness to objectively assess a situation. In the decisive moment, you can choose a response that meets your needs immediately—and in the future. None of us were born with this ability; if you doubt this, spend some time with a 2-year-old. Successful athletes, parents, teachers, and leaders in every field have had to learn this skill. Controlling and directing your emotional state lays the foundation for success, especially when making decisions during emotionally charged times.

## Metabolism 101

It takes energy for you to be you. In every moment of every day, there are millions of chemical reactions occurring inside the cells of your body, all working in concert to keep you alive. Collectively, we call these chemical reactions your metabolism. Everything you do, from breathing to blinking, digesting to sleeping, burns calories. Your resting metabolic rate (RMR) refers to the amount of energy required to keep your body functioning in a state of rest. Depending on your lifestyle and genetics, your RMR may account for up to 80 percent of the calories you burn. This is why people with naturally high metabolisms are able to eat whatever they want without gaining weight. Some of us are less efficient, meaning we have a slower metabolism and find it easier to pack on the pounds. If this is the case for you, it's not an excuse for being overweight.

In a perfect world, we would each be blessed with a metabolism that naturally burns calories at a rate equal to what we're consuming. There would be no need to worry about getting fat or losing weight. In your youth this may have been the case, but as we age our metabolism naturally slows. Compounding the problem, a sedentary lifestyle causes a further reduction of your metabolic rate. Thankfully, your lifestyle and diet, which are directly under your control, influence your metabolism. You get to choose how much you move, what you eat, and what time you go to sleep.

## Digestive System

The average American adult eats 2,000 pounds of food each year. For some of us, that number is considerably more. That's steady work for your digestive system, considering only a third of it ever completes the 27-mile journey to the other end. Thankfully, there's a lot of help along the way. From your mouth to your large intestine to the complex community of microbiota—thousands of different types of bacteria live deep in our digestive tract. You are masterfully designed to efficiently process the foods you eat.

## The Power of Hormones

Hormones are specialized chemical messengers produced by various glands that work together and travel throughout the body, coordinating complex processes such as growth and metabolism. Before we are born, hormones guide the development of our brain and endocrine system, and throughout our lives they control most vital bodily functions—from simple, basic needs such as hunger to complex systems such as reproduction. Even emotions are directly influenced by our hormones. We'll go into more detail in Chapter 5.

## The Power of Sleep

A third of adults don't get enough sleep, and they're paying the price. Apart from "tired" being a bad personality trait, sleep deprivation is linked to a number of serious health issues, including weight gain, depression, anxiety, and decreased physical performance. You may be among the 5 percent of people who function well on very little sleep, but for most of us, a good night's sleep—7 to 8 hours—is essential.

If you're one of the millions of people who have trouble sleeping, here are a few things to try.

- **Keep a consistent sleep schedule.** It pays to have a routine. This is true for your diet, exercise plan, and sleep schedule. Set a bedtime and stick to it. Set your alarm in the morning and get up instead of hitting the snooze button, no matter how tired you are. It can take a few weeks to create a new sleep pattern, but making the effort will not only facilitate weight loss, it will improve every other area of your life.

- **Avoid screens the hour before bed.** Televisions, computers, and phone screens are stimulating and counterproductive to falling and staying asleep. Turn them off and read a book–like the rest of this one.

- **Stay active.** Ideally, you will have worked so hard during the day that by the time 10 p.m. rolls around the only thing you'll feel like doing is sleeping. Exercise contributes to healthy sleep patterns and is an effective way to drain energy. So if you've been lacking in that department, all the more reason to get moving. Check out Chapter 6 for workouts that you can fit into any busy schedule.

- **Don't spend an hour trying to fall asleep.** Your bed is for three things: sleeping, sex, and reading this book. If you're lying there, tossing and turning with a wandering mind, get up and do something distracting. But no matter what time you fall asleep, get out of bed when your alarm goes off.

- **Find a bedtime routine that works for you.** Having a consistent routine in the few hours before bedtime will make falling asleep easier. Winding down your day by relaxing, spending time with family, meditating, reading, or praying will put you in the right state for sleep.

## The Role of Genetics

Obesity has been present throughout human history. But the explosion of cheap, calorie-dense processed foods over the past several decades revealed that a large percentage of the population has a strong genetic predisposition to weight gain. This is unfair, but there's nothing you can do to change it. If that's the hand you've been dealt, you're going to have to pay more attention to your diet than the next guy is.

Brian Foster is a legitimate tough guy–Marine recon soldier, qualified sniper, professional MMA fighter, and outdoor adventurer. He's smart and disciplined, but even when he was in the best shape of his life he still carried fat on his lower abdomen. Some people just cannot achieve a shredded look. Thankfully, Brian is not one to make excuses and didn't let something small, like not being able to achieve a six-pack, stop him from succeeding in all areas of life.

Your genetic code is not a license for self-pity. Acknowledging your genetic makeup empowers you to create achievable goals while accepting who you are. You can achieve results despite your stubborn genes.

## The Importance of Muscle

From a vanity standpoint, muscle looks and feels good. From a health perspective, lean muscle is metabolically active—meaning the more of it you have, the more calories you will burn throughout the day. Muscle improves how insulin regulates blood sugar and preserves strength, which helps prevent chronic diseases such as diabetes and osteoporosis. Many diets can leave you "skinny fat," which means you weigh less, but your percentage of body fat is still high. Don't let this happen to you. Make building muscle a priority as you sculpt your four-pack.

## Your Environment

There is a memorable line from the movie *The Departed*, where Frank Costello says, "I don't want to be a product of my environment, I want my environment to be a product of me." Wonderful line, but for good and bad, we are influenced by where we grew up and even today, your environment continues to influence the person you are. Who do you hang out with? Are they hardworking? Ambitious? Do they inspire you to become a better person? How do you spend your free time? Do these activities contribute to reaching your goals? Research shows healthy team dynamics are essential for success, so put yourself in the right environment to win.

## LEARN FROM THE PROS

Japanese MMA star Ryo Chonan fought in the UFC at a muscular but lean 170 pounds. In the weeks following one fight, he blew up to close to 200 pounds and was basically eating his weight in Popeyes chicken. The difference between how he looked on the scale,

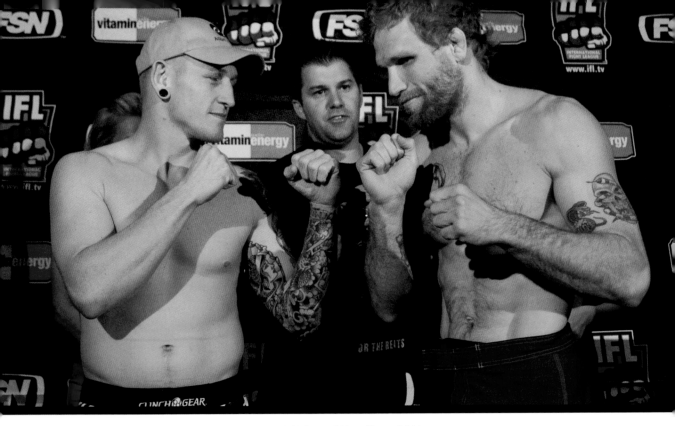

Marine recon sniper? Yes. Professional MMA fighter? Yes. Six-pack? No.

weighing in the day before his fight, and how he looked 2 weeks later was astounding. We personally know many well-known athletes who would never consider doing a photo shoot during much of the year because they don't want to be seen in *off-season* shape. Weight management is also an issue for retired athletes. We call this post-competition syndrome, and it occurs when you no longer have physical goals to work toward. Many retired athletes still eat like they did when training full time. When you factor in age-related hormonal changes and decreased activity due to chronic injuries from years of unhealthy, rigorous training, it's easy to see how significant weight gain occurs in these former gladiators.

What does post-competition syndrome have to do with you? Well, many regular people fall victim to this "no goal/no focus" mindset as well. Gaining 2 or 3 pounds each year doesn't feel significant while it's happening, but fast-forward 15 years and 40 pounds and you've got a real problem on your hands. Joining the 70 percent of overweight adults at risk for all the major health issues affected by the average American diet—heart disease, diabetes, stroke, and premature death—is not something you want to do.

So how do you overcome this doom and gloom? How can you possibly stand a chance against something that often takes down the world's greatest athletes? Should you resign yourself to being a soft mush forever and go crush a steak sandwich? No. Some people develop a reasonably good sense of what works for them early on, while for others it takes a minute to figure out where their sweet spot lies. But there is always a path to victory. It starts with understanding the game, deciding how you're going to play it, and adjusting your approach accordingly.

## NEXT STEP: FIND YOUR BREAKING POINT

We all have one—that place where you can no longer tolerate your current situation. It could be a picture of yourself on Facebook looking way too fat. Maybe you haven't had a date in 10 months, or are unable to get dressed without sweating. Do you want to continue living like this? Are you capable of giving more? It may not be easy to answer these questions, but once you hit your breaking point, you'll uncover resources and motivation you didn't know were available. Here are four steps to get you going.

1.   **Quit feeling sorry for yourself.** Feeling helpless is a debilitating emotion that causes you to miss opportunities because you've become convinced that you are powerless to change. The antidote is discipline. It is a relatively simple muscle to strengthen. Here's exactly what you should do: Start with the dishes—every time you walk by the sink, wash the dishes. When you are finished, you will have done at least one thing right today. Complete this task for a month and magical changes will start to occur. You will have discovered how to establish a new positive habit.

2.   **Break it down.** It's tough to have a compelling vision for the future when you're in a rut. Feeling far from your goals makes it difficult to pick yourself up and get moving. Break a challenge down into manageable chunks and it becomes easier to take that next step. For the next 3 days, can you walk around the block twice? A new you needs to start somewhere.

3. **Harness the power of momentum.** As humans, we fight change as much as possible, which makes getting started the hardest part. So look for the easy way out–find one or two simple changes that won't require much effort, and repeat them! This builds momentum. Once these feel natural, look for other small actions to add to the mix. Chael started by eliminating soda from his diet. Not that big a deal in the grand scheme of things, but it produced results.

4. **Measure yourself.** An objective measurement is a valuable tool to help keep yourself in check. While a scale is not a perfect judge of your progress, it does a better job than just about anything else. Scales are inexpensive, easy to use, and provide impartial feedback. An $8 scale from Walmart may not be the most accurate, so spend a few more dollars to get consistent readings. Have a set point–a red-flag number that triggers an immediate change in your diet.

For those who use food as an antidepressant, this will not be an easy road. You are going to need to identify new outlets to manage stress while developing a bit more mental toughness. Will your life be an inspiration or a warning? If you choose the former, answer this question: What are you going to do about it?

# 3
# LOOK IN THE PAST

## HOW DO PEOPLE GO BANKRUPT? VERY SLOWLY, THEN ALL OF A SUDDEN

## BACK IN THE DAY

Imagine living in a small tribe 10,000 years ago. Infant and child mortality rates were spectacularly high, and survival was never guaranteed. Your days were spent hunting with a spear in hand or foraging for food in the bush. It was under conditions like these that your body became highly efficient at storing energy reserves in the form of fat. Historically speaking, this was an extremely important trait for humans because the risk of starvation was always a real possibility. The more productive you were at storing fat, the greater your chances of survival. The problem with this ancient survival mechanism, though, is that it doesn't turn off in times of abundance. Your hormones, designed to respond in the moment, can't read the future. Unfortunately, what was once an essential trait for survival is now killing us. Why? Despite having easy access to cheap food 24 hours a day, your body still behaves like starvation might be right around the corner. To compound the problem, we are also eating large quantities of food that did not exist 100 years ago, and we're paying a heavy price. The quality and quantity of the foods that make up the average American's diet have contributed to an increase in heart disease, stroke, diabetes, and cancer. And from a purely aesthetic point of view, that thick layer of fat covering your glorious abs isn't sexy.

Our genetic traits have been overwhelmed by advancements in food technology and distribution. Modern, large-scale food production rapidly changed fundamental aspects of our diet, especially over the past century, and pushed many of us well past our genetic limits. With a digestive system unable to cope, a new era of diseases has been ushered in. Cardiovascular disease will account for over 38 percent of all deaths in America this year. Fifty-nine million people suffer from high blood pressure, and 11 million have type 2 diabetes. The second-leading cause of death in the United States, behind heart disease, is cancer, and approximately one-third of all cancer deaths are due to poor nutrition—including obesity. So given our current situation, it's worth our time to explore how our ancient ancestors lived, since they were free from many of the ailments that plague us today.

With the proliferation of lifestyle-related diseases, it's easy to wax nostalgic about the good old days. Recently, an idyllic view of cavemen diets has become quite popular. But there was no standard caveman fare. A caveman living in Alaska had a much different diet than his cousins in the Fertile Crescent. Humans are the most successful creatures on the planet for one reason—we are adaptable. From the arctic tundra to equatorial rain forests to remote islands, we have conquered every continent and successfully adapted to their unique climates and natural resources. Even today, in areas of the world where food scarcity affects a large percentage of the population, birth rates are still high. We don't just survive. We thrive. So why have so many people struggled with the onslaught of processed foods? For some, the tipping point has been reached. Even the incredible adaptability of the human body has its limits.

In human history, there have been two significant periods where technological advancement changed how we eat. The first food revolution occurred somewhere between 8,000–10,000 years ago, when cultivating crops and raising domesticated animals first began. Farming introduced vegetables and grains, and protein from livestock provided a more secure and steady food supply. Although these foods were not a significant part of the menu during our hunting-and-gathering years, it doesn't necessarily mean they are bad for us. Many have been consumed for thousands of years without causing obesity and diabetes.

The real problem came about much later. As food technology rapidly advanced during the industrial revolution, the nutritional makeup of our diet was significantly altered, particularly in the past 50 years. It has reached the point where a major percentage of our modern diet is composed of foods that have never been encountered before in human history. In 2005, the *American Journal of Clinical Nutrition* published a study that stated 72 percent of the modern Western diet consists of dairy products, refined sugars, vegetable oils, and alcohol. None of these foods were found in pre-agricultural diets. Those ancient grains and oils were given a makeover and the results are not pretty. The quality of life for an increasingly large percentage of our population is declining as a direct consequence of the foods we are eating. It's not difficult to narrow down a list of suspects. Let's take a look at six recent additions to our diet and explore how they contribute to our weight problems.

## 1. Dairy Foods

Wrangling wild animals and having them stand still long enough to be milked is not an easy task. It turns out there are very few qualified candidates for the job. Have you ever tried to milk a giraffe? It's tough. They are quite tall and known to be excellent kickers. Of the 6,000 species of mammals that produce their own milk, we depend on *one* for 97 percent of our dairy products—the cow. Before cows were domesticated, when our ancient ancestors were done with mommy's milk, that was it.

In the grand scheme of human history, we haven't been consuming dairy for very long, and intolerance is common. Despite the new version of the food pyramid from the USDA called "MyPlate," which recommends that we consume dairy, there is no evidence that drinking milk prevents bone fractures. Countries reporting the lowest dairy and calcium consumption also report the lowest rates of osteoporosis. In fact, dairy may increase the risk for fractures in women by 50 percent, according to a Nurses' Health Study. There's also research suggesting a connection between dairy and prostate cancer. One more thing: Almost all the dairy we do consume has been exposed to high heat, a process called pasteurization. In an effort to make this product safe, many nutrients and enzymes are destroyed, changing the nutritional properties of this food. Something to think about.

## 2. Cereals

Have you ever tried to harvest wild cereal grains? We hear it's quite hard to do. But admittedly, we're not survivalist types. The difficulty of harvesting grains is one reason why they were not included in the diet of our ancient ancestors. Another reason is that of the 9,000 species of grass around the world, only 35 have been cultivated as edible cereals. Historically, if you lived in a part of the world where these grasses did not grow natively, you were out of luck. Obviously, grains would not have been part of your diet.

When it comes to grain consumption, one invention changed everything. In 1831, 22-year-old Cyrus McCormick made the final adjustments to his father's invention: the mechanical reaper. This innovative machine automatically cut, threshed, and bundled grain while being pulled through a field by horses. Until this point, this backbreaking work was done by hand with a scythe, which limited the amount of grain a farmer could grow.

Eventually mechanical reapers caught on, allowing farmers to produce significantly more food—especially corn.

While advances in farming have increased food production necessary to feed a growing world population, they have also fueled the processed food industry and changed how livestock, poultry, and fish are raised for human consumption. Today, 50 percent of cereal grains grown in the US are used to feed livestock in commercial feed lots. Almost all grains consumed in the US are highly processed and refined, which negatively impacts the nutritional characteristics of the food. Even milling healthy grains into flour changes the speed at which our bodies digest these carbohydrates and contributes to a spike in blood sugar. Nutritionally, a slice of white bread is not the same food as an equal amount of whole, sprouted ancient grains.

## 3. Refined Sugars

Before sugar production escalated, it was relatively difficult to eat excessively sweetened foods. Sure, there was honey, but that was seasonal and did not make up much of the ancient diet. And don't forget those pesky bees. In 1700, the average person consumed 4 pounds of sugar per year. In the late 1970s, chromatographic fructose enrichment technology made high-fructose corn syrup commercially viable. As the processed food industry grew, so did our consumption of refined sugar. Ryan spent several years in a sugar cane–growing region of Australia and witnessed the challenges a modern cane farm has to navigate. Genetically engineered seeds, designed to withstand a heavy onslaught of chemical fertilizers, are now the norm and new crop diseases are common. According to the USDA, the average American will consume 150 to 170 pounds of sugar this year. As this global science fair project continues to play out on a massive scale, the results are not looking good.

## 4. Refined Vegetable Oils

Refined vegetable oils are a relatively recent addition to our diets. The first oil cultivated for human consumption was olive oil, around 6,000 years ago. Sesame oil appeared in the Mediterranean basin and India by 1137 BC, and in South America the Aztecs were producing peanut oil long before European settlers arrived in the 15th century. Until the late 19th century, the only edible oil-bearing crop grown in Europe was the olive.

The biggest change in oil consumption resulted from technological developments in the 1800s that allowed commercial oil production to scale. Mechanically driven steel expellers and hexane extraction increased oil yields, and new manufacturing procedures such as hydrogenation transformed vegetable oils into margarine. Vegetable oils such as rapeseed, soy, and sunflower not available before 1900 underwent rapid production increases in the 1950s and by the late 1980s had become the dominant oils found in world markets. These newly formulated fats were inexpensive and used in most processed foods, contributing to the rise of modern lifestyle diseases such as obesity, heart disease, and diabetes.

## 5. Salt

The first evidence of salt mining dates back to around 6000 BC in China. Today 75 percent of our salt consumption comes from processed foods, while only 15 percent comes from adding salt to our meals while sitting at the table. We all respond somewhat differently to sodium. It contributes to high blood pressure for some and has very little effect on others. If you are looking to reduce salt intake, start by eliminating processed foods. Pay attention to nutrition labels found on the packaging of the foods you eat. Aim to keep your salt intake between 1,500 and 2,300 milligrams per day.

## 6. Fatty Domesticated Meats

Commercially raised animals produce different meat than their wild, free-roaming cousins. In wild animals, body-fat percentages vary–by species, age of the animal, and time of year. When food is plentiful in the summer, excess calories are stored as fat. As seasons change and food supply becomes limited, fat is depleted to help the animal make it through lean times. Domesticated animals, fed large amounts of grain, produce meat with dramatically different fatty acid profiles, with more saturated fat and considerably less high-quality essential fatty acids. As corn prices have increased over the past several decades, it's not uncommon for cows to be fed candy like Skittles and ice cream sprinkles–these can be purchased for half the price of corn and the sugar helps fatten up the cattle.

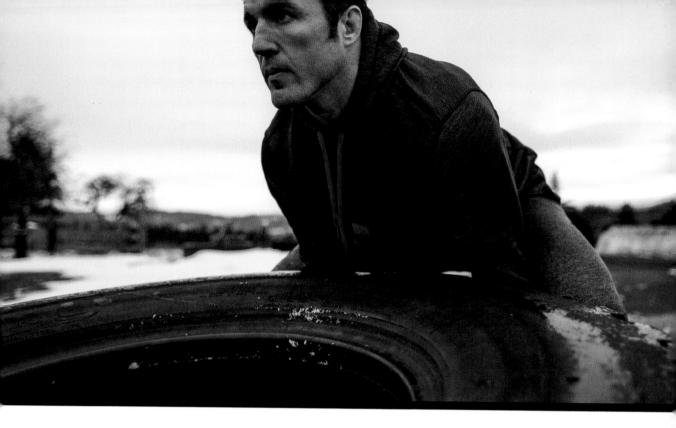

Animals raised in a feedlot also exercise considerably less than wild animals, which impacts the overall health of the animal and the meat it produces.

Raising cattle on grass works best for producing happy cows and healthy meat, but it's much too slow for large commercial cattle producers. Before 1850, all cows were organic, pasture-fed, free-range animals. In the second half of the century, feedlots were born from technological advances in agriculture and transportation—particularly increased corn yields, the expansion of railroads, and refrigerated freight cars. Before this time, access to "fresh" meat was a challenge in the city, since animals had to be slaughtered and butchered in the area the meat was going to be sold. Live cattle were sent on a perilous journey by train to local slaughterhouses. It wasn't uncommon for cows to lose 100 pounds or even die along the way. Now it was possible to ship a finished, packaged product to major metropolitan areas with limited meat supplies thousands of miles away. These changes made scaling the nation's beef supply more economical and efficient.

By the 1950s, the commercial feedlot era was in full swing and by 1968, the largest had grown to accommodate 100,000 cattle. Cows gain a tremendous amount of weight—up to 6 pounds per day—eating high-grain diets in feedlots, and the physical condition of these grain-fed animals can best be described as obese. A telltale sign of feedlot beef is white fat that is firm in texture, due to high amounts of saturated fat.

Up to 97 percent of the beef consumed in the United States is the product of a feedlot, where cows have been given a steady supply of antibiotics to combat disease in their crowded, dirty living quarters. Today a modern feedlot can produce a cow ready for slaughter in 14 months, sometimes less. But over the past decade, there has been a growing number of ranchers raising and finishing cows on the fields where they were born. Experts predict that the organic beef market may represent 30 percent of the entire market in the future. Even though there's a long way to go, it's easier than ever to find healthier meat options.

In 2005 a team of researchers from universities in the United States, Australia, and Sweden published a paper in the *American Journal of Clinical Nutrition* that examined how the evolution of the food we eat fundamentally altered seven essential elements of our diet. These dietary changes have led to worldwide public health crises and provide a good place to start when looking for opportunities to improve the way we eat.

## Glycemic Load

The concept of glycemic load was developed in 1997 as a way to measure how quickly specific foods raise blood sugar. Refined carbohydrates—grains and sugar—have significantly higher glycemic loads than natural fruits and vegetables. The massive shift to more refined carbohydrates and fewer vegetables in a typical Western diet adversely affects metabolism and insulin resistance. It also chronically elevates blood sugar levels while setting the stage for modern-day inflammatory diseases such as obesity, heart disease, diabetes, and cancer. Choosing carbohydrate foods with a low glycemic load such as nuts, legumes, fruits, and vegetables will help reset your system.

## Fatty Acid Composition

Our modern diet has significantly affected not only the quantity of fats we are eating but, more importantly, the type of those fats. High intake of refined vegetable oils, found in the average Western diet, alters the dietary ratio of omega-6 to omega-3 essential fats. Traditionally these fats were consumed in equal amounts, but now it's not uncommon for people to eat 15 times more omega-6 fats than omega-3s. The problem is that consuming large amounts of omega-6 fats, especially those found in refined vegetable oils, promotes inflammation. Since coronary artery disease, cancer, stroke, diabetes, and arthritis have roots in inflammation, these poor-quality oils put you at risk. The fix is an easy one: Stay away from processed foods and add an omega-3 supplement, and you're on your way.

## Macronutrient Composition

Carbohydrates, fat, and protein make up the majority of the foods we eat. According to the *American Journal of Clinical Nutrition*, today's Western diet averages 52 percent carbohydrates, 33 percent fat, and 15 percent protein, and many of these calories come from refined carbs and unhealthy processed oils. The increased consumption of these processed foods represents a major shift in modern diets and is a significant risk factor in degenerative diseases such as diabetes, arthritis, Alzheimer's, and heart disease. Although it is not possible to determine exactly what our ancestors ate for dinner 10,000 years ago, studies of modern hunter-gatherers show higher protein intake (19 to 35 percent of energy) and lower carbohydrate (22 to 40 percent) consumption.

## Micronutrient Density

Processed foods, including refined sugars and oils, are essentially devoid of vitamins or minerals. As our diets have become overloaded with these unhealthy foods, nutrient-dense ones have been pushed out. This reduces the amount of micronutrients in our diet, putting us at risk for vitamin and mineral deficiencies. Yes, there are foods fortified with vitamins and minerals, but there is something about the balance of nutrients in natural foods that's difficult to replicate in a lab. Increasing the amount of whole foods and especially vegetables will help restore balance. If you don't like to eat your veggies, try juicing them.

## Acid–Base Balance

Everything we eat has an effect on the body's biochemistry. After eating, digesting, absorbing, and metabolizing a meal, nearly all foods release either acids or bases into the

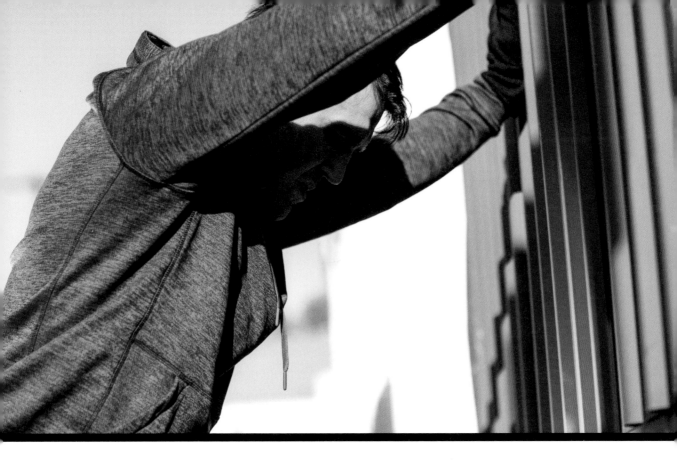

bloodstream. Proteins such as meat, poultry, fish, eggs, cheese, milk, and shellfish are acid-producing. Basic, or alkaline-producing, foods include fresh fruit, vegetables, tubers, roots, and nuts. Legumes are generally neutral. The typical Western diet produces more acid than base, which leads to chronic low-grade metabolic acidosis, a condition in which the body produces excess acid. As we age, this negatively impacts kidney function. The diet of our ancestors was net base-producing. By increasing our consumption of alkaline foods and reducing our intake of acidic foods, we are able to reduce our chances of developing osteoporosis, muscle atrophy, kidney stones, hypertension, and exercise-induced asthma.

## Sodium–Potassium Ratio

Potassium is essential for maintaining pH levels and plays an integral role in blood pressure regulation. Optimum ratios of dietary sodium and potassium are important for a number of reasons, including protection from high blood pressure and heart disease. As we mentioned earlier, modern humans consume a significant amount of salt. Unfortunately, at the same time our diet has also become deficient in potassium, leading to an imbalance between these two micronutrients. Eliminating processed foods is the easiest way to alter your sodium–potassium ratio, since they tend to be high in sodium and low in potassium.

The standard American diet averages about 2,500 milligrams a day of potassium, while the recommended daily allowance is 4,700 milligrams. Leafy greens, nuts, apricots, salmon, and mushrooms are high in potassium; meeting the daily requirement is easily accomplished with Four-Pack Revolution recommended foods (see Chapter 4). Correcting the sodium–potassium imbalance is straightforward with a few additions to your diet.

- Eliminate processed food, a major contributor to an unbalanced sodium–potassium ratio.
- Drink green veggie juices. Although the fiber is removed during the juicing process, you're able to consume larger volumes of veggies and micronutrients, including potassium.
- Add potassium-rich foods to your diet, such as avocado, cooked spinach, lima beans, broccoli, Brussels sprouts, asparagus, and winter squash.

## Fiber Content

Our grandparents were more concerned about eating fiber than our generation is, and Grandma was right. Today most of us don't consume nearly enough fiber–on average, 12 grams per day, while our ancestors consumed over 40 grams. Fresh fruit has twice the fiber of whole grains, and non-starchy vegetables contain almost eight times the amount. Fiber found in fruits and vegetables slows the process of digestion, helps reduce appetite, and increases satisfaction after a meal, while most importantly feeding the colony of microbiota that lives in your digestive tract. Eating fiber also has the added benefits of lowering the bad (LDL) cholesterol and preventing constipation.

Increasing fiber intake to 30 to 40 grams per day by consuming more vegetables is

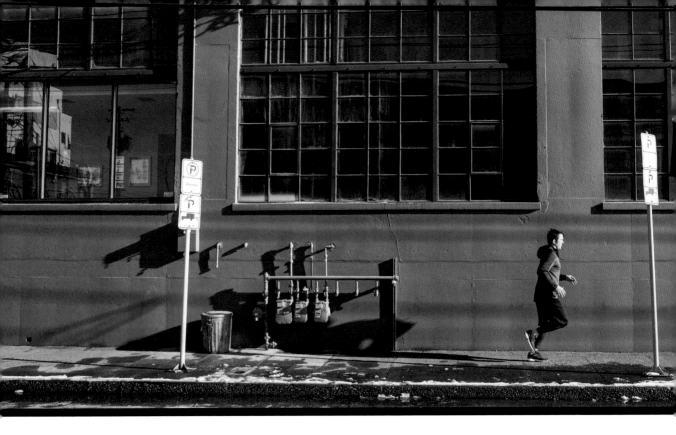

not hard to do. A diet that includes regular consumption of legumes and non-starchy veggies will easily get you there. An avocado alone has 10 grams, and a cup of chickpeas (garbanzo beans) has 12 grams. If one of your meals contains either of those ingredients, you're likely to hit your daily fiber goal.

## LOOK TO THE FUTURE

As you look to the future, a basic understanding of our dietary history along with an awareness of your resources, capabilities, and limitations leads to better decision making and healthier eating habits. It's similar to the stock market—if you understand what factors cause stock prices to rise or fall, you can reap rewards. Successful, long-term weight loss rarely involves one fix. Just as heart disease does not result from just eating too much sugar, weight loss is influenced by a combination of nutritional, lifestyle, and genetic factors.

What about our ancestral heritage? There are valuable insights from the ultimate old-school diet. But the extremists yearning for caveman life need to eat a doughnut from time to time. The human body is an incredible machine—adaptable, creative, and resilient. There is a solution in which modern living and traditional diets can peacefully coexist. While 10,000 years does not make up a significant percentage of the history of mankind, culturally it's a very long time. We are more than just eating machines. Food is woven into the fabric of our lives. For some of us, our genetic makeup allows us to eat modern foods with limited negative consequences. For others, the impact is catastrophic. This is why you need to learn what works for you, both culturally and physiologically.

For those of you who have had enough of the restrictive fad diets, demonization of food, and unrealistic expectations about how you should look, your suspicions are correct: It's impossible for you to look like a fitness model. Don't fall into the trap of believing a magic bullet will fix your problems. Leave those for the late-night infomercials. You need a better solution. In the next few chapters, we will cover everything you need to create an ideal diet, including how to visually judge the perfect portion size; exactly which carbohydrates, proteins, and fats are best to eat; and how to excel once a week with a System Reset meal that will neutralize any cravings—all while creating the four-pack of your dreams. So what's the plan? Anticipate failure. Lower your expectations. Create lasting results. The Four-Pack Revolution will show you how.

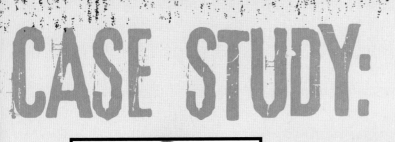

# CASE STUDY:

## CASEY
### (AGE 31)

**I like keeping my life simple.** There are fewer decisions to make. This approach worked for my diet as well. Being a routine-oriented single male, I would meal-prep on the weekends and put a week's worth of breakfasts and lunches into separate plastic containers. This usually took less than 30 minutes. When I didn't make time to prepare food in advance, I always had a quick go-to meal that would be ready in a few minutes. A bag of washed spinach, a can of beans, and some leftover chicken was an easy, reliable meal to fall back on, and using different spices added variety.

The first 2 weeks were a challenge, as I felt hungry earlier than usual, but adding a snack toward the end of my workday helped take the edge off. This allowed me to eat my lunch a little earlier in the day and avoid getting hungry in the late afternoon. Limiting my carb intake, especially in the morning, also had a big effect. Once my body got used to it, I noticed a major boost of energy and didn't need three cups of coffee to get through the day.

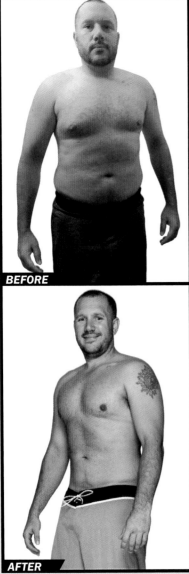

BEFORE

AFTER

**JAN 5:** 227 lb, stomach 44 in, waist 38 in
**FEB 5:** 217 lb, stomach 41 in, waist 36 in
**MAR 5:** 210 lb, stomach 39 in, waist 36 in

## PLAN

- 3 to 4 meals a day (breakfast, lunch, snack, dinner)
- 60 percent veggies for each meal
- 20 percent protein for each meal
- 20 percent beans for each meal
- 16 oz water upon waking up
- 40 oz water throughout the day
- Minimal calories through fluids—only water/tea/coffee
- No calories through sauces (dressings, ketchup, BBQ sauce, etc.)

## BREAKFAST

- Chopped bell peppers, onions, cauliflower rice, frozen mixed veggies
- Plain grilled chicken breast or lean turkey
- Black beans or mixed beans
- Dry seasoning (changed daily)
- Eggs, egg whites (if I felt like I needed more protein)
- Avocado (a couple times a week)
- Coffee with no sugar and a small amount of cream

## LUNCH

- Spinach
- Grilled chicken breast
- Black or mixed beans
- Mustard and balsamic vinaigrette for dressing
- Homemade tea (no sugar) or kombucha tea

## SNACK

- Cauliflower rice, frozen mixed veggies
- Lean turkey*
- Black or mixed beans

  *Grilled with various dry seasonings*

## DINNER

- Cauliflower rice, frozen mixed veggies
- Fish (salmon or any white fish)
- Black beans or mixed beans

## SYSTEM RESET

- Eat anything I want: pizza, pasta, sushi, candy, etc.
- Still avoid drinking lots of calories

## EXERCISE

**First month: limited exercise**

- Mon, Wed, Fri: body-weight squats, pushups (20–30 in the morning and evening)
- Sat or Sun: hiking

**Second month: increased frequency**

- Mon–Fri: Body-weight squats, pushups (30–40 in the morning and evening)
- Sat or Sun: hiking

**Third month: increased duration**

- Mon, Wed, Fri: body-weight squats, pushups (20–30 in the morning and evening)
- Tues, Thurs: jog 3–5 miles
- Sat or Sun: hiking

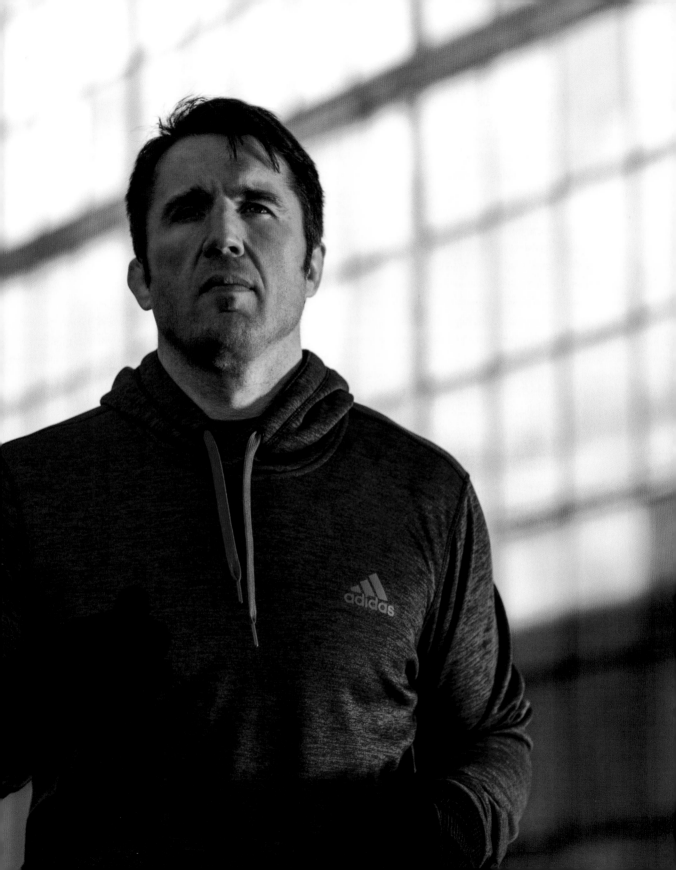

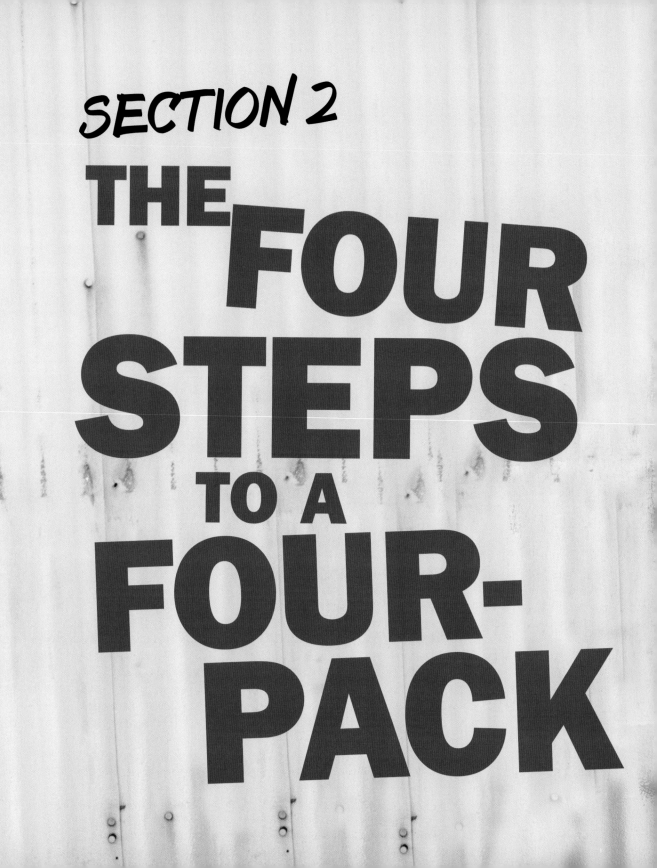

SECTION 2

# THE FOUR STEPS TO A FOUR-PACK

# 4
# FOUR-PACK MEAL COMPOSITION

**I WAS 28 YEARS OLD WHEN I HAD MY FIRST GLASS OF WATER. EVERY TIME I TELL** people that, they laugh or think it's a joke, but I'm not kidding. My coaches used to tell me how important it was to drink water, and they were not alone. Every diet I can remember always emphasized the importance of drinking water. It didn't matter if you were on Weight Watchers or some plan your meathead buddy recommended. There was even a diet called the water diet. But I never believed this advice had any merit. As a wrestler, I was always trying to lose water weight, so why would I possibly drink more? I compared it to fat: If I'm trying to lose fat, I'm not going to eat fat. At the time, this all made perfect sense to me.

Just to clarify: When I say I never drank water, I'm not counting gym class at school or wrestling practice, where we only had a water fountain. But I never had a glass or bottle of water, not one time. Pepsi was my number one choice. It wasn't just me. My parents didn't drink water. My sister didn't drink water. None of us did. Every day after wrestling practice, my dad would take me across the street to 7-Eleven and hand me a dollar bill. I'd go inside while he waited in the truck and buy a Big Gulp for 99 cents. With no sales tax in Oregon, I'd leave the penny on the counter and walk out like a gangster. Every day, that was our routine.

Here's how I came to realize the importance of drinking water. I was traveling to Las Vegas to fight Trevor Prangley in the UFC. Prior to my trip, I heard Ivan Salaverry, a talented fighter whom I looked up to, say, "If you guys ever fly anywhere, make sure you drink a lot of water on the day that you fly. It will help with jet lag." When I landed in Las Vegas, I had 18 pounds to lose in 3 days in order to reach the 185-pound limit of my weight class. Drinking water 3 days before weigh-in went against my philosophy, but for some reason Ivan's words resonated with me.

Sitting in my hotel room at the Hard Rock, I started drinking water. Every time I peed, I'd drink even more. When I woke up the next day, I'd lost 4 pounds and I couldn't believe it. This worked so well that for my next few fights, I repeated the process. When I landed on Tuesday, the beginning of fight week, I'd start drinking water–lots of it. I didn't measure how much I drank, but this simple change in my routine made losing weight for my fights much easier. Cutting weight is a terrible experience, and I was all for anything to make it easier.

Over the years, I found a gallon of water per day worked best for me. But instead of waiting until fight week to start hydrating myself, I begin 30 days prior to my fight. One gallon–that's a little over 8 pounds of water–every day. Usually, after the first day I lose 2 or 3 pounds; the next day, 1 or 2 pounds. My weight loss slows down after 3 or 4 days, but overall I feel better and find it easier to eat healthier as well.

There is a downside to drinking large amounts of water, with the most severe side effect being water intoxication, which can be deadly. When the body has too much water relative to its salt level, significant neurological problems or death can occur. Don't be a dummy who tries to drink multiple gallons of water a day thinking it's a miracle cure. Go slow. Test and see what makes you feel best.

For most of us, the challenge of staying properly hydrated throughout the day takes some planning. You must have water with you at all times–in your car, at work, at home. A water bottle should be a permanent accessory. When I give this advice to my high school wrestlers, I tell them, "Take a water bottle to class, keep one in the car, and have one close by at home. Sipping small amounts regularly works best." Another challenge that comes with drinking more water is having to pee constantly. To put that in perspective, I pee one time in the middle of the night, every single night, 365 days a year. When I am drinking a gallon a day, I go four times. That may not sound like a big deal, but it is because it disrupts your sleep. Depending on my schedule, there are times I don't drink a full gallon a day. When I'm in business meetings, I can't get up to use the bathroom every 30 minutes. So on those days I'll make adjustments.

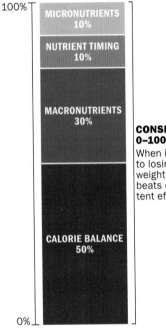

100%

MICRONUTRIENTS
10%

NUTRIENT TIMING
10%

MACRONUTRIENTS
30%

CALORIE BALANCE
50%

0%

**CONSISTENCY
0–100%**
When it comes to losing weight, nothing beats consistent effort.

Eating can't be an all-or-nothing proposition. Long-term success comes by creating balance. While nutrition advice is easy to come by, it can be overwhelming trying to navigate the latest research and applying this information in a way that works for you. So let's keep it simple. We're going to break down what we consider to be the four pillars of good nutrition, list them in order of importance, and explain each in detail. With these four pillars as your foundation, you can craft a plan for success. It doesn't have to be perfect, just sustainable. A balance between healthy living and enjoying what life has to offer.

## THE FOUR PILLARS

### Pillar 1: Calorie Balance (50% of the equation)

In some ways, the ratio of the types of food on your plate is more important than what you actually eat. It's very difficult, without the use of expensive lab equipment, to know the exact calorie count of a meal, but if you take one thing from this chapter, understand this:

It's easy to learn how to gauge the macronutrient ratio and portion size of the food on your plate. This is the first step in creating a balanced meal, and 40 percent carbohydrates (the more non-starchy vegetables, the better), 30 percent protein, and 30 percent fat is a good place for most people to start.

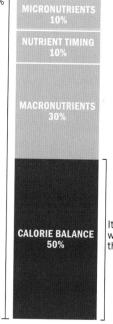

### SERVING SIZE VERSUS PORTION SIZE

A serving size is the amount of food recommended on a nutritional label. A portion size is how much food you choose to eat at one time. Sometimes these are equal, but other times they're not. Once you have established the correct ratio of macronutrients, portion size is what determines if you will lose or gain weight. In most Western cultures, the average portion size has increased significantly over

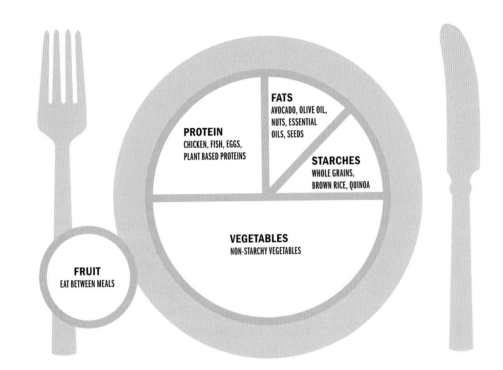

FATS
AVOCADO, OLIVE OIL, NUTS, ESSENTIAL OILS, SEEDS

PROTEIN
CHICKEN, FISH, EGGS, PLANT BASED PROTEINS

STARCHES
WHOLE GRAINS, BROWN RICE, QUINOA

VEGETABLES
NON-STARCHY VEGETABLES

FRUIT
EAT BETWEEN MEALS

the past 20 years. For those who have been to Japan, you know that a "large" is usually equivalent to a "small" in the United States. Numerous studies have shown that when food tastes good, people will consume whatever is put in front of them and, if offered seconds, the answer will usually be yes. Understanding portion size makes it easier to stop eating before you're full.

## VISUALLY IDENTIFY PROPER PORTION SIZES FOR EASY DECISION MAKING

Very few people can successfully count calories. It requires a combination of brainpower, maintaining a food journal, and luck. Most people underestimate how much they eat and overestimate how much they move. An easy solution is to learn to visually identify the optimum portion that delivers the desired percentages of protein, carbs, and fat.

Once you understand how to balance the food on your plate and determine the proper portion size, the next step is to focus on the quality of the foods you're eating.

| HAND SYMBOL | EQUIVALENT | FOODS | CALORIES |
|---|---|---|---|
| | FIST<br>1 CUP | RICE, PASTA<br>FRUIT<br>VEGGIES | 200<br>75<br>40 |
| | PALM<br>3 OUNCES | MEAT<br>FISH<br>POULTRY | 213<br>110<br>204 |
| | HANDFUL<br>1 OUNCE | NUTS<br>RAISINS | 170<br>85 |
| | 2 HANDFULS<br>1 OUNCE | CHIPS<br>POPCORN<br>PRETZELS | 150<br>120<br>100 |
| | THUMB<br>1 OUNCE | PEANUT<br>BUTTER<br>HARD CHEESE | 170<br>100 |
| | THUMP TIP<br>1 TEASPOON | COOKING OIL<br>MAYONNAISE,<br>BUTTER<br>SUGAR | 40<br>35<br>15 |

## Pillar 2: Macronutrients
## (30% of the equation)

Protein, carbohydrates, and fat make up the bulk of your diet and supply energy in the form of calories and essential nutrients. These macronutrients are what most people think about when deciding whether a food is healthy. For years, fat had a bad reputation. Then carbohydrates came into the crosshairs. Now even protein is often misunderstood. But not all carbs are bad and not all protein and fats are good. So let's explore each macronutrient to find out what's really going on.

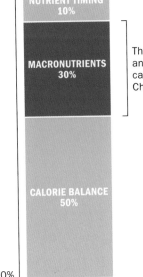

There are good and bad proteins, carbs, and fats. Choose wisely.

### PROTEINS

If you want to lose weight, look better, and control food cravings, then protein is the single most important nutrient for you to consume. Protein boosts metabolism, reduces appetite, and influences several weight-regulating hormones. While protein may be used for energy under some conditions, its main role involves tissue maintenance, production, and repair. Proteins, like excess carbohydrates, can be converted to and stored as fat.

The eternal question surrounding protein has always been "How much do I need?" The answer is that there's no one-size-fits-all approach. Your age, weight, body-fat level, and activity all play a role in the ideal amount of protein you need to consume each day. Taking in 25 to

**PROTEINS**

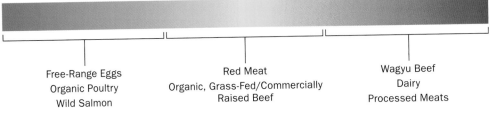

Free-Range Eggs
Organic Poultry
Wild Salmon

Red Meat
Organic, Grass-Fed/Commercially
Raised Beef

Wagyu Beef
Dairy
Processed Meats

30 percent of your daily calories as protein is a good place to start and has been shown to be effective for weight loss. If you are on a 2,000-calorie-a-day diet, 30 percent amounts to 150 grams of protein.

### Protein Timing

Eating protein with each meal throughout the day as opposed to one large protein meal helps regulate and stabilize several weight-regulating hormones, including the hunger hormone ghrelin. This effect leaves you feeling satisfied after a meal and therefore helps you consume fewer calories overall. Another benefit to protein is that it requires more energy to digest than carbohydrates or fat do. This is called the thermic effect of food. (More on this in a bit.)

## CARBOHYDRATES

Carbohydrates are the most talked about topic in nutrition. Now that fats are no longer villainized, the focus has shifted to carbs, and for good reason. From Atkins to the Paleo Diet, the no-carb or low-carb trend is dominating the nutritional marketplace. Cheap, easily accessible, carbohydrate-rich foods are a major contributor to everything from tooth decay to obesity. As a culture, we've become addicted to beverages loaded with sugar and snack foods made from processed carbs. The sugar industry knew the dangers of refined carbohydrates a long time ago. *JAMA Internal Medicine* recently published an article that exposed the Sugar Research Foundation, an industry group that began funding research at Harvard University in the 1960s to downplay the risks of sugar and instead point the finger at fats. Internal documents from the organization revealed they wanted to "refute" any connection between sugar and the development of heart disease. It was good for business to convince the public to eat more sugar and less fat.

Some people can eat carbs without gaining any weight, while others seem to gain 6 pounds after eating one plate of pasta. So you must adjust your carbohydrate intake based on how your body reacts to these foods. For most of us aiming to lose weight, reducing carbohydrate intake is important, especially processed carbs (more on that next). If you are significantly overweight or have struggled with your weight for years, reducing carbohydrates in your diet can have a profound effect on your weight loss and overall health.

## CARBOHYDRATES

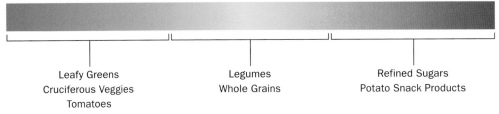

| Leafy Greens | Legumes | Refined Sugars |
| Cruciferous Veggies | Whole Grains | Potato Snack Products |
| Tomatoes | | |

### Recommended Carbohydrate Food Sources

Apart from a System Reset meal or special occasion (yes, it's okay to have a piece of birthday cake), certain carbohydrates should be avoided altogether. The list is long and includes

# A TALE OF TWO CARBS

**When you think of potatoes, it is natural to think of potato chips, like Pringles.** Potatoes are a vegetable and come from the earth, so why wouldn't a thin slice of a potato be a good thing to eat? Especially Pringles, those perfectly shaped, crispy, salty delights. Well, not everything that comes from nature is good for you, and not every ingredient in a Pringle is from a potato. In fact, in July 2008, lawyers from Procter & Gamble, the company that owns Pringles, successfully argued in the London High Court that Pringles contained only 42 percent potato and that the final product was a substance not found in nature. (This was to get out of paying a 17.5 percent tax on potato snacks, by the way.)

### Pringles

**The life of a Pringle starts in the dirt.** Probably a field in Idaho. Growers start with seed potatoes and harvest between August and October every year, depending on the type of potato being grown. During the growing season, fertilizers and pesticides are used to reduce disease but organic potatoes have restricted allowances as to what can be used. While potatoes can be processed into Pringles at the time after harvest, most are kept in humidity- and temperature-controlled storage for processing during the remainder of the year. Fresh potatoes are delivered to supermarkets, while the rest are trucked to processing plants, where they are used to manufacture everything from french fries to potato flakes.

If you have ever eaten a Pringle, you have probably noticed that they do not resemble a potato—or taste like one either. The ingredients are processed with the help of modern food science to achieve their addictive qualities. Most potato-based snack products are created from a processed form of potatoes—either dehydrated potato flakes or flour. The processing involves inspection and peeling, cutting the potatoes into slabs, blanching in water to swell the starch cells (this toughens them so they resist rupturing, which would cause the substance to become sticky) before being steam-cooked and mashed. Next, this potato mash is dried until it winds up looking like a large piece of paper, before being milled to the desired particle size.

potato chips, fruit juices, sodas, and other snack foods, along with the enormous caffeinated drinks topped with whipped cream and flavored syrups proffered by prominent national coffee chains. These refined carbs have had all of their nutritional value stripped away and are often referred to as "empty calories," but there's nothing empty about them. These products are linked to overeating, inflammation, diabetes, and heart disease and are a major cause of resistance to vital hormones that control how much we eat, the rate at which we burn calories, and the strength of our food cravings. We'll discuss these critical hormones, insulin and leptin, in Chapter 5.

If you are overly sensitive to pasta, bread, and rice (meaning they easily make you gain weight), your best bet is to switch to beans in place of those foods. Legumes are inexpensive, they taste great, and there are myriad ways to prepare them. Along with

To make Pringles, the finished potato flakes are sent to another food manufacturing facility where they are combined with wheat starch, corn, and rice flour. Dough conditioners, water, and highly processed shortening are added before the mixture is kneaded into a dough. Other ingredients can include sweeteners such as maltodextrin and dextrose, monosodium glutamate (MSG), disodium inosinate, disodium guanylate, sodium caseinate, modified food starch, monoglyceride and diglyceride (processed fats), autolyzed yeast extract, natural and artificial flavors, malted barley flour, and cheddar cheese.

Since a Pringle is highly processed, many of the starch cells are broken down during manufacturing. This causes digestion to occur rapidly, which is why highly processed potato-based products have an immediate effect on blood sugar levels. All carbohydrates are sugar and are broken down into the same form—glucose. When your blood sugar rises, the hormone insulin steps in to escort glucose into your cells while excess sugar left in the bloodstream is converted to fat. The more this cycle occurs, the less effective insulin becomes, and diseases such as diabetes begin to take root.

### Garbanzos

A can of chickpeas, also called garbanzo beans, takes a very different path from the soil to your plate. Like Pringles, garbanzos start in a field, but this is where the similarities end. After being harvested and delivered to a processing facility, chickpeas are sorted, classified by size, and separated from damaged grains or other foreign material with vibrating separation equipment. Soaking overnight hydrates the beans and also removes phytic acid and other enzyme inhibitors that may cause gas and heartburn. This enhances both digestibility and nutrient absorption. The final step is canning, where each filled can is steam-heated to 250°F for an hour before cooling and having a label applied. If you were to buy dried garbanzo beans at the store and cook them at home, the end result would be almost identical.

When chickpeas enter your digestive tract and are absorbed into your bloodstream, they elicit a much different response from your blood sugar than Pringles do. It is like the difference between 20 drunk teenagers crashing your house party and having George Clooney show up. Nutritious foods like garbanzos, high in fiber and protein, stabilize blood sugar and leave you feeling satisfied after a meal.

green vegetables, they should be your go-to carbohydrate foods. If you are still finding it difficult to lose weight after making this switch, reduce the amount of beans in your diet and increase the amount of non-starchy leafy greens. Your job is to experiment and find what works best for you.

For some, eliminating sugar and other refined carbohydrates will be the most difficult step in the weight-loss journey. Not to worry. As your taste buds return to normal over the first few weeks your cravings will diminish. Anticipate this challenge, stay hydrated, and focus on the positive benefits coming your way. These feelings will pass. Stick it out; it will be well worth the effort. Try a "no added sugar" 30-day challenge. It's a great exercise to build awareness about the foods you're eating, and you may be surprised by the results.

## FATS

Fats have gotten a bad rap over the years. The controversy started in the 1950s when it was observed that countries whose citizens consumed elevated amounts of saturated fat had higher death rates due to heart disease. Researchers mistakenly blamed saturated fat as the sole cause, and it took a long time for fats to shed this terrible reputation as a nutrient to be avoided at all costs. But it turns out we need fats in our diets. They make food taste better, help slow blood sugar spikes after meals, and protect our vital organs while influencing immune function, reproduction, and other aspects of basic metabolism.

There are three main types of dietary fat found in the foods we eat: saturated, mono-unsaturated, and polyunsaturated. The unique chemical configuration of each type of fat determines how it is used in the body. Like carbohydrates, not all fats are equal. The quality of the source and the type of processing greatly influences their health properties. For example, refined, processed oils are some of the most dangerous foods found in our diet. They dominate supermarket shelves and often have a clear, yellow color. You most likely have a bottle of refined vegetable oil in your kitchen cupboard right now. Do yourself a favor and throw it out! Healthy sources of fats include nuts, seeds, fatty fish, extra virgin olive oil, avocados, and organic, naturally raised animal products. Pay close attention to how oils are processed—exposure to heat, light, or air during manufacturing, distribution, and storage can turn healthy fats rancid.

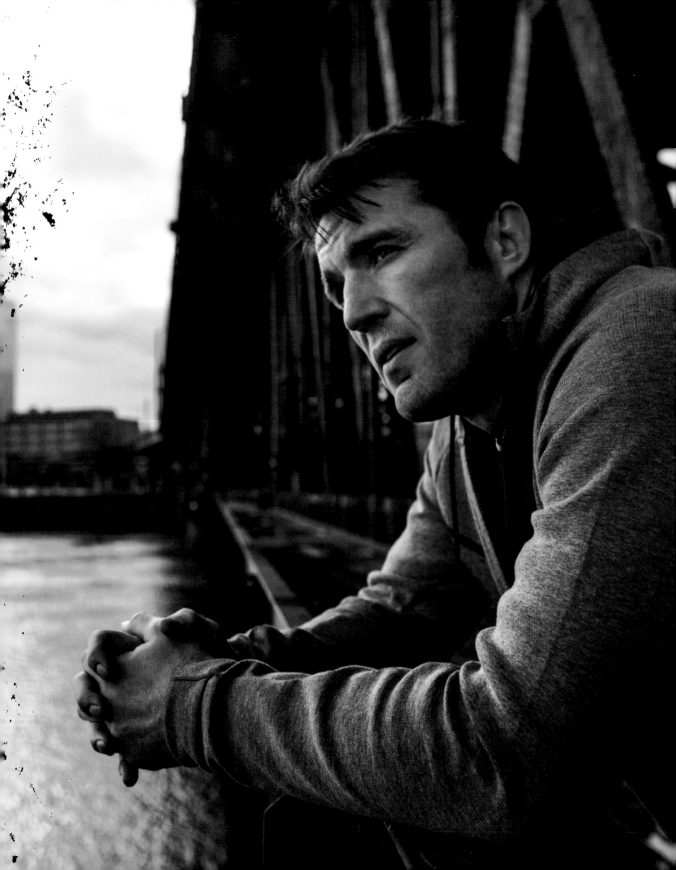

**FATS/OILS**

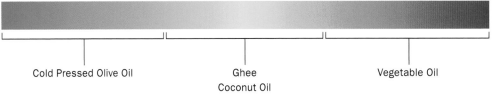

Cold Pressed Olive Oil        Ghee        Vegetable Oil
Coconut Oil

### Saturated Fats

Due to their chemical nature, saturated fats, with the exception of coconut and palm oils (tropical oils), tend to be solid at room temperature. Most of the saturated fat we consume comes from animal products—meat and dairy. Diets high in saturated fats and low in consumption of whole plant foods contribute to an unhealthy balance of mono- and polyunsaturated fats. This combined with excess processed carbohydrates sets the stage for the development of inflammatory conditions such as obesity.

Palm and coconut oils, used in many processed foods, are often industrially refined rather than used in their native forms. If you choose to consume these tropical oils, make sure they are unrefined (e.g., whole coconut oil or extra-virgin, cold-pressed coconut oil). Since the majority of our dietary saturated fats come from animals, look for pasture-raised organic meat. The fatty acid profiles of these foods will be healthier than those raised in large, commercial farms.

### Monounsaturated Fats

These important dietary fats (oils) are liquid at room temperature but solidify in the refrigerator. In whole food form, healthy monounsaturated fats are found in nuts, seeds, olives, and avocados. They lower LDL cholesterol (aka the "bad" cholesterol) and increase HDL cholesterol (aka the "good" cholesterol) while developing and maintaining cells and supporting your immune system. Eaten in place of unhealthy fats, monounsaturated fats also help people with type 2 diabetes manage their blood sugar.

### Polyunsaturated Fats

Polyunsaturated fats are divided into two classes: omega-3 and omega-6 essential fatty acids. They are considered essential because our bodies cannot synthesize them, so they must be obtained from the foods we eat. It is not recommended to cook with polyunsaturated fats since these volatile oils are easily damaged when exposed to high heat. They are also sensitive to air and light, so it's important to store them in a cool, dark place. Lastly, fresh oils are best, so pass on buying in bulk because they perish over time.

**Omega-3 Essential Fatty Acids.** These essential fats are among the most important nutrients in your diet. Necessary to support a healthy immune system, omega-3s are also associated with a reduced risk of heart attack and stroke, improved brain function, and decreased inflammation.

There are three omega-3 fatty acids.

- ALA (alpha-linolenic acid): found in plant-based sources (hemp, flax, walnuts)
- DHA (docosahexaenoic acid): found in marine products
- EPA (eicosapentaenoic acid): found in marine products

EPA and DHA are critical omega-3 fatty acids used as the building blocks for hormones that control immune function, blood clotting, and cell growth. If you eat fatty fish like salmon a few times a week,

*(continued on page 60)*

## COMMERCIAL OIL FOOD PROCESSING

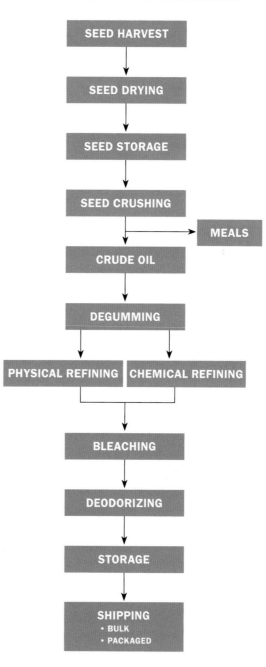

# A TALE OF TWO OILS

**Most of the fats and oils you've been eating have been heavily refined in modern food processing plants.** These oils are altered for several reasons. Manufacturers need a product that, in addition to being edible, is bland in flavor and odor, clear in appearance, light in color, stable to oxidation (meaning it has a long shelf life), and suitable for frying. While oils with these characteristics make it possible for companies to be profitable while fitting into the infrastructure of modern food distribution, there are downsides. The refining process strips all the nutrients from the oil and creates a product that wreaks havoc in our body.

## Vegetable Oil

**That plastic bottle of vegetable oil sitting on your shelf went through many steps to get there.** Seeds used to make cooking oils are dried to less than 10 percent moisture, cleaned of foreign matter and de-hulled. The kernels are ground and steamed before the oil is extracted in a screw or hydraulic press. What's left over is a pressed cake that is flaked for later extraction of residual fat with solvents such as "food grade" hexane. Hexane may sound familiar to you because it is a by-product of the refining of crude oil. Hexane is also found in industrial cleaning products, textile production, and rubber manufacturing. Sounds great, right?

Here's the next stage of the refining process.

1. **DEGUMMING:** The first step is to remove gums that are naturally present in the oil. These gums are responsible for a loss of oil yield and easily decompose, darkening the oil due to their thermal instability.

2. **NEUTRALIZING:** The free fatty acids found in the oil are treated with caustic soda and converted into soaps before being removed in a centrifuge.

3. **BLEACHING:** The oil is bleached with a special clay at high temperature to remove pigments, trace metals, and oxidation products. After the bleaching clay is filtered out, the remaining oil is much lighter in color and has an extended shelf life.

4. **DEODORIZING:** This process uses steam to remove natural compounds from oils that may affect taste and stability. Many of the compounds that are removed are nutritionally valuable and provide cardiovascular and anti-inflammatory benefits as well as protection against certain cancers.

Thankfully, this is not the only way to process oils. There are small producers using traditional methods that, combined with modern science, produce some of the best-tasting, healthiest oils ever made.

## Organic Olive Oil Production

**Apollo Olive Oil takes a very different manufacturing approach.** In its quest to make the world's finest olive oil, it was the first company in the United States to press olives in a vacuum. Why is this important? When exposed to heat, light, or air, oil begins to break down in a chemical reaction called oxidation. This is why antioxidants are important—they prevent this process from happening. You may have seen ascorbic acid on a nutritional label before. Ascorbic acid is also known as vitamin C, which is an antioxidant added to foods to prevent oxidation.

Apollo also takes a different approach when planting their olive trees. They allow for space between each tree, not like the high-density planting technique used in large-scale farming. This leads to healthier trees that don't require pesticides to protect them from disease. They also harvest ripe olives by hand, which is more expensive but ensures that the skin of the olive is not broken or bruised during the process, which would lead to oxidation of the oils. Oxidation creates "free radicals" that have been proven to increase the risk of heart disease, stroke, and cancer. Have you ever cut an apple and noticed the inside starts to turn brown after a few minutes? That's oxidation in action. Any exposure to heat, light, or air speeds up this process, and causes healthy oils to turn rancid.

The olive fruit used by Apollo is pressed within 4 hours of being picked to ensure there is minimal degradation. After a wash, the olives are mixed in a vacuum to separate the oil from the pulp. In this step, the fresh oil is at a high risk for oxidation which is why Apollo elects to separate their oil in a vacuum. The absence of oxygen protects the oil, improves its taste, and preserves its natural health properties. Next, a decanter is used to separate the oil from the pomace. While most olive oil producers use a centrifuge to separate the oil and water, Apollo uses mechanical filters. While the yield is lower and the process is more labor intensive, the resulting taste and nutrient values are much higher. For Apollo, these practices are a trade-off. Their product does not have as long a shelf life, and they are not able to scale up their production like large manufacturers. They have made a conscious choice to remain small while delivering the highest quality oil possible.

If you're curious how the olive oil you buy in the grocery store has been processed, give it a sniff. Processed oils can often smell rancid. You may not even realize the oil you're smelling is off because that's how all the oil you've ever consumed has smelled. Pay attention to musty, vinegary, or metallic odors. Oils that start to turn rancid will often have a smell that resembles crayons, putty, or old peanuts. Some processed oils may not have much smell at all, but this is a sign that the oil has been refined in the same large-scale way we outlined earlier. A taste test will tell you even more: Fresh olive oil leaves a clean taste from the healthy polyphenols still present in the oil; refined oils leave a greasy sensation on your mouth, which is another sign of oxidation. Different olives produce different flavors. Some oils may have a bold, peppery taste, while other varieties may be subtle with aromas such as fresh cut grass, almond, or artichoke. Unfortunately, almost all the oils sold in supermarkets are highly processed and can have potentially damaging effects on your body.

According to the USDA, people in 1960 spent an average of 17.5 percent of their income on food. This fell to 9.6 percent by 2007, and continues to trend downward. It's cheaper to eat now than it ever has been, and with 7 billion people on our planet, this is a good thing. But there's a sacrifice that comes with the drop in food prices, and you have to decide if the risks are worth it. Healthy oils are essential for optimum health. Spending an extra $10 every few months on high-quality oil is an easy change that can move you in the right direction.

In a perfect world, our food supply would come from our own backyards, but this isn't a realistic approach. Feeding everyone on the planet would be an impossible task without modern food production. But you are an individual, and you get to choose the role refined or natural foods play in your life. If you don't live in an area where healthy foods are easily accessible, there are many sources of unrefined, natural foods available to anyone with a PayPal account and an internet connection. Making small changes is a great way to enhance results, and changing your olive oil is a quick, easy win.

(continued from page 57)

you're probably getting enough of these essential oils. While ALA is supplied by vegetarian sources such as walnuts and flaxseeds, it must be converted to EPA and DHA by the body. Unfortunately this conversion isn't very efficient, so if you're not a fan of fish, consider adding a fish oil supplement to your diet to ensure that you're getting enough EPA and DHA.

**Omega-6 Essential Fatty Acids.** These essential dietary fats are needed for normal growth and development and, most importantly, brain function. They help regulate metabolism, support skin and hair growth, and work to maintain the reproductive system. But too much of a good thing can be harmful. Today, most of our intake of omega-6s comes in the form of processed vegetable oils, not whole foods. In 2007, CNN's Dr. Sanjay Gupta reported that according to the National Institutes of Health, refined soybean oil, which is high in omega-6s, is the most consumed oil in the United States, accounting for up to 10 percent of the total calories in the standard American diet. It's inexpensive to produce and is added to many processed foods. An overabundance of dietary omega-6 fatty acids contributes to inflammation in the body and disrupts the healthy balance with their cousin, omega-3s.

### Omega-3 to Omega-6 Ratio

The ratio of the foods you eat applies to individual oils as well. The ideal ratio of omega-6 to omega-3 essential fatty acids is 1:1, as was the case for most of human history. Due to the sheer volume of refined vegetable oil in our diets and low intake of foods high in omega-3 oils, the average ratio today is more like 15:1. This is one of the most important dietary inadequacies to correct. Lowering the ratio of these two essential oils to close to 1:1 significantly reduces your risk of developing a host of preventable inflammatory diseases.

## Pillar 3: Nutrient Timing
## (10% of the equation)

Nutrient timing is based on the premise that when you eat, not just what you eat, is important. Athletes rely on nutrient timing to maximize the nutritional benefits of food to build and repair their bodies. If you've ever made the effort to eat breakfast within 30 minutes of waking or made a post-workout protein shake, then you are familiar with this concept. Properly timing your meals throughout the day stabilizes blood sugar and tames cravings. Having healthy go-to meals ready is a must. It takes a little planning and preparation, but the results are worth it.

There's more leeway in nutrient timing than originally thought, and it turns out your body can adapt to a number of different food timing strategies. But this is still a valuable consideration since, for some people, specific meal timing can be very effective. At the very least, it helps organize your day and makes keeping a consistent meal schedule easier.

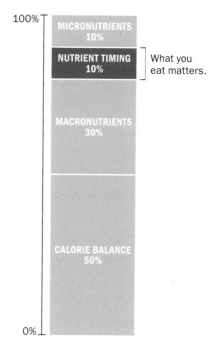

## WHAT ABOUT BREAKFAST?

We've all heard that breakfast is the most important meal of the day, and for most people it is. After fasting overnight, chances are you're hungry when you roll out of bed. So eat! You have a long day ahead of you, and the right fuel will help get you going. But the standard modern breakfast of processed meat and refined carbs doesn't help the cause. Consider how your first meal of the day will affect your mindset and performance until lunchtime. You can prevent a mid-morning crash with 20 to 30 grams of protein, a small serving of slow-digesting carbohydrates, some vegetables, and healthy fat. Eggs cooked in olive oil or ghee alongside a cold-brew coffee protein shake blended with spinach is an inexpensive, easy-to-prepare example that fits the bill. You should experience an increase in your energy level and mental function while promoting fat burning throughout the day.

What if you don't like to eat first thing in the morning? Then don't! Just be prepared to eat a Four-Pack meal whenever your body feels ready. A muffin and sugar-laden coffee drink won't cut it.

## PRE- AND POST-WORKOUT MEALS

All of us should expect to see results if we are going to make the effort to work out, and timing your intake of protein and carbohydrates can make a difference. If it's been a while since you have eaten, a small meal 1 to 2 hours before exercise will help you perform better. But keep in mind, training on less food may help you burn fat and improve insulin sensitivity, so don't overdo it. Dr. John Ivy, a leading researcher in carbohydrate timing, has published many studies showing the potential benefits of controlling when you consume this important macronutrient. Post-workout is the best time to eat higher carbohydrate meals. The effect of insulin escorting blood sugar into the cells will be highest, allowing your body to process dietary carbohydrates more efficiently than at any other time.

Here are some guidelines to get you started.

1. **Never go more than 5 hours without food.** Three to 4 hours is ideal. Our goal is to keep blood sugar steady throughout the day. Spacing out well-balanced meals helps control hunger and cravings and will improve your mood. You are probably not much fun to be around when you're hungry.

2. **Eat four to six times per day.** You can vary this by having six smaller meals, three meals and two snacks, etc. Experiment and see what feels best. You'll also need to remain flexible when life gets busy. Sometimes it is impossible to eat six small meals throughout the day, so three meals and two snacks might work better for your schedule. The key is not waiting until you are overly hungry to enjoy a meal. Planning goes a long way. Know where you can find healthy food when you are out, or remember to bring prepared food with you.

3. **Avoid snacking.** Snacking has become a hobby for many people. The middle aisles in every supermarket have been taken over by processed snack foods. Manufacturers pay big money in the form of "slotting fees" to have their products displayed in this prime real estate for one reason—there is much demand. Snacking is often a result of boredom or stress, and the best way to avoid these extra calories is to stay busy. A focused mind cannot be distracted by potato chips.

## Pillar 4: Micronutrients (10% of the equation)

Micronutrients, also known as vitamins and minerals, are only needed in minuscule amounts but are vital to producing enzymes and hormones used throughout the body. Since these micronutrients are not produced in our bodies, they must be derived from our diet, which is why we recommend that you focus on eating vegetables, legumes, nuts and seeds, lean meats, and fish. Relying on whole foods for these nutrients is the best way to make sure your body absorbs them properly.

100%

**MICRONUTRIENTS 10%**

Essential vitamins and minerals play a central role in metabolism and health.

**NUTRIENT TIMING 10%**

**MACRONUTRIENTS 30%**

**CALORIE BALANCE 50%**

0%

## WATER

Water is the most commonly overlooked nutrient. But how much water should you drink? Eight glasses a day. Says who? Why eight glasses and not nine? Or seven? This is one of those blanket recommendations that doesn't make a lot of sense. Would a 300-pound football player working out in full pads on a hot day in August need the same fluid intake as a 55-year-old office worker?

Most people don't consider water a nutrient—but it's the single most important component of your diet. It is so vital that you can't live without water for more than a few days, and proper hydration is directly linked to optimum health and performance. There are several studies that show even mild dehydration significantly impacts your physical and cognitive abilities.

The two best ways to monitor your hydration needs are simple: thirst, and the color of your urine. If you are thirsty, drink some water. It's not rocket science. Many people confuse thirst with hunger. If it's only been a few hours since your last meal and you find yourself staring into the refrigerator, drink two glasses of water instead. There is a good chance your hunger will disappear for an hour or so. When you go to the bathroom, take notice of the color of your urine. If it's clear or light yellow, you are properly hydrated. Dehydration causes your body to hold on to water, and your urine becomes concentrated and dark yellow in color.

Your hydration needs vary depending on diet, time of year, and exercise intensity. So get into the habit of carrying a water bottle with you and sip regularly. Since many people are dehydrated before they begin working out, drink 12 to 16 ounces of water 20 minutes prior to exercising. If you are still looking for an exact number of how much to drink, start with 2 liters per day, or about eight glasses.

## GETTING YOUR NUTRITION ON TRACK
## (OR BACK ON TRACK)

Now that you understand the basics, making educated food choices should be easy. The days of wondering what and how much to eat are over. What's left is discovering how to fit these changes into your lifestyle. Even if you have started a "diet" before and didn't reach or maintain your target weight, remember that you are never more than one decision away from getting back on track. Here are four areas to focus on.

1. **Fix deficiencies:** It's easier to begin by adding missing items than to eliminate specific foods. Start by making sure you're getting enough water, protein, essential fats, and micronutrients. Find different food sources that work with your body and move you toward your four-pack goal. Make sure you enjoy your meals, or your chance of long-term change will decrease significantly. There are lots of options if you are willing to keep an open mind.

2. **Self-test:** Ultimately, you are the one in charge. Test different foods or a new recipe (see Chapter 9) and see how you feel. You need to eat every day for the rest of your life, so when deciding what to eat, use these four questions to help guide your food choices.
   - Will this food strengthen my body?
   - Will this meal help me lose weight?
   - Is this something I'll enjoy eating?
   - How will I feel after this meal?

3. **Fine-tune:** Life is always changing, so you'll need to make adjustments along the way. Look for opportunities to shave calories whenever possible. Use water in your protein shake instead of milk. Instead of three eggs in your breakfast, use two eggs and two egg whites. Leave the cheese off your dinner salad. These changes might not seem like much, but over the course of a month, small adjustments lead to measurable results.

4. **Be adaptable:** Life can be crazy, and the only certainty is uncertainty. Develop the ability to remain flexible and adjust your approach when things are not working. This develops confidence and builds emotional strength.

## System Reset

For many, just the thought of permanently eliminating certain unhealthy foods is enough to make any dietary change seem miserable. The good news is you don't have to. In fact, we encourage a meal every week in which you eat anything you'd like. This isn't a "cheat meal," which implies something negative. A better description is a *System Reset*. These meals can have positive effects, so why not embrace and enjoy them? Let's set aside any guilty food emotions for a moment and consider some of the benefits to eating our favorite "forbidden" foods once a week. A System Reset meal provides a mental break and gives you something to look forward to. If you are treating yourself right by eating Four-Pack foods and exercising the majority of the time, your body can absolutely handle one unhealthy meal each week. Enjoy it!

### SYSTEM RESET MANAGEMENT

Since most of the foods found in these meals are unhealthy, managing a System Reset becomes crucial. The first consideration is timing—once a week is fine, once a day is not. Just like a river ecosystem, your body is designed to process a certain amount of pollutants without disrupting its natural balance. But there is a tipping point where those toxins overload the system and it can no longer protect itself. Second, our aim is to minimize any negative effects that come with a gluttonous meal. Eating a small amount of protein 45 minutes prior to your meal can help you instinctively eat less, and scheduling your

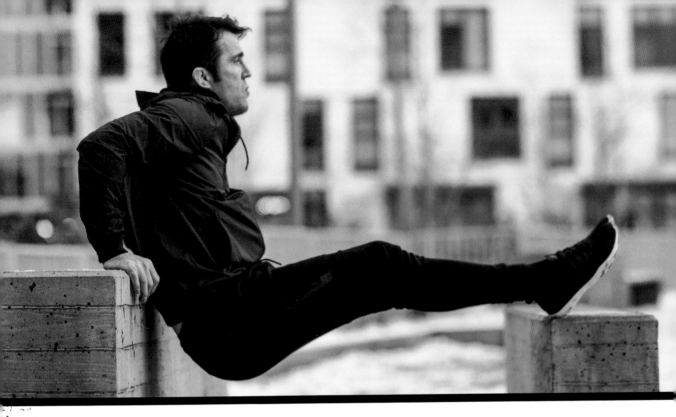

hardest workout on a System Reset day will put you in the strongest position to process the food. Lastly, learn how to keep a System Reset meal in its place. Eating is an emotional topic, and it's not uncommon for all sorts of unusual thoughts and negative emotions to be linked up to specific foods. One meal is nothing to be ashamed of, so enjoy the food for what it is and move on.

## OVERVIEW

As you can see, the basics of what to eat are pretty simple. By keeping the four pillars in mind, you can leverage food to change your body composition instead of falling victim to poor or uninformed dietary choices. With a little planning and experimentation, you will easily create delicious go-to meals that support your four-pack goal.

Cutting back on bread, pasta, potatoes, and sugar will help control your blood sugar, and slow-digesting carbs like chickpeas provide all of the fuel you'll ever need. Choosing healthy proteins and fats along with essential fatty acids will leave you feeling satisfied and keeps your metabolism humming along. Use the portion size chart on page 49 to keep your calories within a healthy range and you're good to go. And lastly, once a week go for it—eat whatever you'd like and enjoy it!

Remember:

- Drink lots of water: up to a gallon per day. Adjust your fluid intake to account for excessive sweat loss during long workouts. A good rule of thumb is that your urine should be mostly clear (unless you're taking vitamin supplements, which can affect the color).

- Put your fork down several times during the meal and stop eating before you're full. You can always find more food if you need it. Try this—talk to the person sitting across from you.

- Avoid eating late in the evening. But if you're hungry, a small carbohydrate meal may make falling asleep easier.

- Eat lots of vegetables with every meal. Veggies are loaded with phytonutrients and fiber that are required for your body to function at its best. Get creative with how you consume them: Put them in your protein shake, toss them on the grill, or use leftovers in your morning omelet.

- Consume 20 to 30 grams of protein per meal (about 30 percent). Protein keeps your metabolism moving along, increases lean muscle mass, and reduces body fat.

- We all need carbohydrates. Our individual levels of carb sensitivity and lifestyle dictate exactly how many complex starches we need, and there are lots of healthy choices, from quinoa to sprouted grain breads and pastas. Save the sugar, processed carbohydrates, and that plate of fettuccine from your favorite Italian restaurant for a System Reset meal.

- Legumes/beans are a perfect food. High in protein, fiber, and complex starches, there are numerous varieties that are inexpensive, easy to prepare, and taste great. Throw a can of great northern beans, a few handfuls of spinach, and a little olive oil in a pan, add some leftover chicken from dinner last night, and you have a perfect Four-Pack lunch ready in minutes.

- You need fat to perform at your best. Avocados, nut butters, seeds, and fish oils are all excellent sources. Around 30 percent of your calories should come from fat. Create a healthy balance between saturated and mono- and polyunsaturated fats for optimum nutrition. Start by correcting any omega-6 and omega-3 fatty acid imbalances first.

- Develop the habit of preparing food in advance. This may be the single most effective strategy for maintaining a healthy eating plan. Having a protein shake available at the end of your workout or healthy snacks in the office will help you stabilize your blood sugar and keep your day running smoothly. Leftovers provide the fastest way to throw together a healthy meal in minutes.

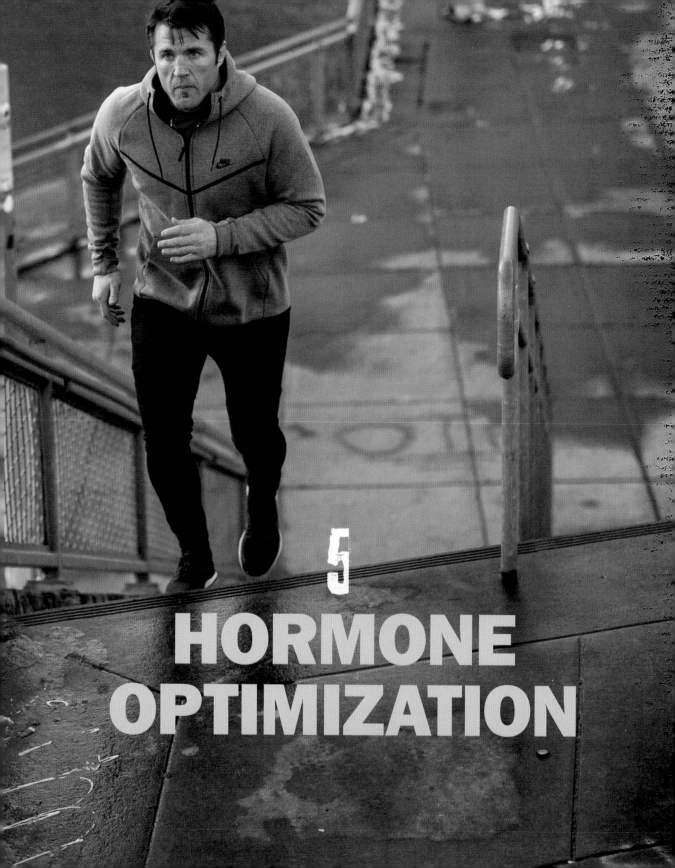

# 5
# HORMONE OPTIMIZATION

**A**H, HORMONES. THESE FASCINATING CHEMICAL MIRACLES WERE RESPONSIble for turning you into an asshole at age 13, and they still direct and influence every aspect of your life today. Produced by various glands, hormones travel throughout the body working together to coordinate complex processes such as growth and metabolism. Before we are born, they guide the development of the brain and the endocrine system, and throughout life they control most of our vital bodily functions, from basic needs such as hunger to complex systems such as reproduction. Even emotions are directly influenced by our hormones.

An epic display of the power of hormonal imbalance comes from our good friend Heath Sims. Heath was an amateur wrestler who burst onto the national stage at 18 years old, placing second in the 1990 USA World Team Trials. For the next decade, he sacrificed as he pursued his dream to one day become an Olympian.

First, a little background on how you make an Olympic team in wrestling. During an Olympic year, you need to enter the national tournament. This is an open tournament, meaning anyone can sign up; you could enter this year if you wanted to. Those who manage to place in the top eight are invited to compete in the Olympic trials (usually held 3 or 4 weeks later).

In the spring of 1996, with the national tournament just weeks away, Heath was feeling confident. Years of training had refined his technique, and competing overseas against the world's best taught him how to remain calm and perform under pressure. It wasn't fun dropping 20 pounds to reach the 149.5-pound weight class limit, but Heath had done it many times before and always returned to a healthy 170-plus pounds within a day of making weight.

Although Heath wrestled well and placed third, for some reason, a day after the competition, he ballooned up to 196 pounds with pitting edema in his legs. His legs and feet were so swollen that when you pressed your finger into his ankle, the indentation would remain for several seconds.

There are serious consequences for dehydrating yourself, as Heath regularly did. When your body senses a sudden change in hydration, your blood vessels, brain, and digestive system work overtime to maintain fluid levels. Hormones that control fluid retention influence the brain and the kidneys, and their normal physiological function becomes compromised. Not exactly ideal for a world-class athlete just weeks away from the Olympic trials.

Panic set in as the scale flashed 196 pounds. This was 20 pounds heavier than Heath had ever been, and there wasn't time to lose enough weight to reach the 149.5-pound limit for the trials. His only option was to move up a weight class to 163 pounds. This just added to his stress and stacked the odds further against him, as the wrestlers he'd be competing against in that weight class naturally weighed 15 pounds more than he did. But even at this heavier class, Heath still struggled to lose the weight. The combination of calorie deprivation, dehydration, and intense training threw his body so far out of whack that he was unable to regain control in time, and he failed to make the Olympic team.

There is a happy ending to this story. With some adjustments to his diet and training, Heath went on to place eighth at the Olympic Games in Sydney four years later. It is a good reminder that our failures are not fatal and that for those willing to keep an open mind, there is always a way to turn things around. At the very least, this is a cautionary tale against crash diets.

Our bodies produce approximately 50 different known hormones, many of which are involved with metabolism, muscle growth, hunger, and weight. Appreciating how four specific hormones influence your weight will go a long way toward your understanding of how to harness the power of your body to burn fat and build muscle. Once you see how easy it is to direct these hormones with food and exercise, you'll be more inclined to take action. Stick with us—there is some science coming up—but after reading this section, you'll know how to leverage these weight management hormones instead of fighting them like Heath did.

## CORTISOL

Cortisol is most often associated with infomercials and belly fat. But there is so much more to this power hormone. Cortisol helps with memory formation and reduces inflammation. It influences salt and water balance and helps control blood pressure. When you're under stress or in danger, a surge in cortisol and adrenaline (see page 72) triggers your body to burn calories from carbohydrates instead of fat. Bodily functions that are not critical in the moment, such as the immune and reproductive systems, shut down to conserve energy. You have a threat to face; making babies can wait—now it's time to kick some ass. As you may imagine, cortisol is intended to be relied on only for a short period of time. Once you're out of danger, cortisol levels naturally decrease. No one needs to be in fight mode 24/7—it's a great way to lose friends and infuriate people.

Long-term stress is a totally different animal because it causes cortisol to remain elevated. Unfortunately, in the presence of cortisol, insulin's ability to escort blood sugar (glucose) into cells is compromised. And as your blood sugar level rises, so does your risk for obesity, diabetes, and heart disease.

Chronically elevated cortisol affects energy levels and suppresses immune cells, making you more susceptible to illness. Constant stress, coupled with overproduction of cortisol and adrenaline, also negatively impacts your thyroid gland. Gone unchecked, this can lead to fatigue, weight gain, depression, allergies, joint pain, headaches, and digestive problems. Intense hunger and food cravings are also common, and testosterone production can decrease over time. Yikes! Cortisol is a magical chemical that gives you the power to take on any problem—or it can take your daily stress (real or imagined) and convert it into a physical illness. A side benefit to the Four-Pack Revolution plan is that everything we recommend in this book will help manage your cortisol levels. So take a deep breath and keep reading.

## ADRENALINE

Adrenaline is another hormone that's called on when stress levels rise. Its release triggers the body's fight-or-flight response, causing air passages in the lungs to dilate to provide your muscles with the oxygen needed for quick action. At the same time, your blood vessels contract to redirect blood toward the major muscle groups, as well as your heart and lungs. Adrenaline reduces your body's ability to feel pain and causes a noticeable increase in strength and performance, as well as heightened awareness. You may have heard stories about mothers performing feats of incredible strength when their children are in danger, like lifting up a car. It's not a bite from a radioactive spider or being exposed to a gamma ray that causes this superpower—it's adrenaline.

You are miraculously designed to handle life-threatening situations and could not survive without this hormonal response. Just don't spend a lot of time here. Chances are you are not much fun to be around when you're in high stress mode, and over time your

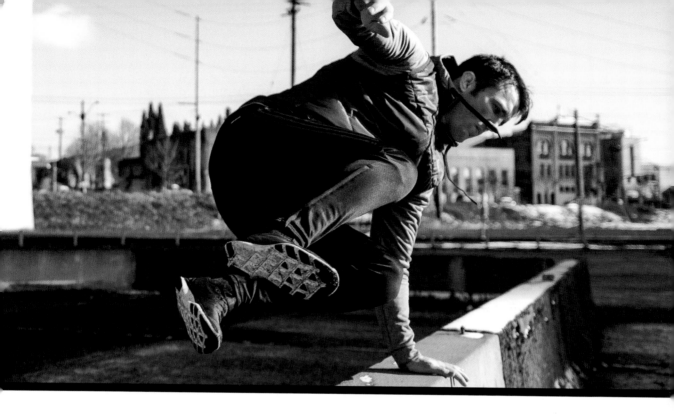

body and relationships will pay the price. When adrenaline is released during times of mental or emotional stress (instead of real physical danger), it can leave a person feeling restless and irritable. But never mind that—too much adrenaline circulating in your blood can also lead to heart failure. Stress management, prayer, meditation, adequate sleep, and herbal teas can all lower the amount of adrenaline in your bloodstream. Learning to chill out is a valuable life skill for a number of reasons.

## LEPTIN

You may think that gaining weight is just about excess calories and a lack of exercise and willpower. However, modern obesity research tells a different story. Scientists have identified a hormone called leptin that has a tremendous impact on your appetite. This "master" hormone, produced in the body's fat cells, regulates body weight and is often called the satiety or starvation hormone.

Leptin targets an area in the brain called the hypothalamus. One job of the hypothalamus is to recognize when the body has enough energy stored or when, instead, it needs more fuel. When functioning properly, this mechanism keeps you from starving or overeating. But unhealthy diets and sedentary lifestyles have led many to become resistant to leptin. For these people, the brain doesn't receive the message that they've had enough to eat. They continue to experience the physical sensation of hunger even when excess calories have been consumed.

Willpower alone is not strong enough to overcome the urge to eat when your brain thinks you are starving. It's very difficult to lose weight under these circumstances, and the problem doesn't stop there. In response, your metabolism slows, fewer calories get burned, and your energy level decreases. Leptin resistance is now believed to be a leading cause of weight gain.

## What Causes Leptin Resistance?

**Inflammation:** Foods such as processed meats, sugar, and trans fats cause inflammation in the body, affecting blood vessels, the heart, the brain, and muscles. Inflammatory messengers, recognized by your brain, specifically the hypothalamus, cause a resistance to leptin.

**High levels of leptin:** Since leptin is produced in the body's fat cells, more fat cells equals more leptin. It would seem logical to assume that elevated levels of leptin would be beneficial since its job is to tell your brain that you've had enough to eat, but unfortunately the opposite is true. Elevated leptin causes the brain to become resistant to its messages, creating a vicious cycle that causes people to eat more and gain weight.

## How to Reverse Leptin Resistance

Body fat, especially around your belly, is a key indicator that you have become resistant to leptin. The first step toward turning this around is to add anti-inflammatory foods to your diet, such as the ones recommended in the Four-Pack plan. And exercise helps to build lean muscle mass and increases your metabolism while improving the action of other important hormones, including insulin.

## INSULIN

This powerful hormone's primary job is to regulate the amount of nutrients circulating in the bloodstream. Rising blood sugar levels trigger insulin to be secreted into the bloodstream, allowing muscle, fat, and liver cells to absorb glucose to be used for energy.

### Here's How Insulin Works

When you eat a meal containing carbohydrates, the amount of sugar circulating in your blood increases. So let's say you eat a bowl of pasta. Cells in your pancreas recognize

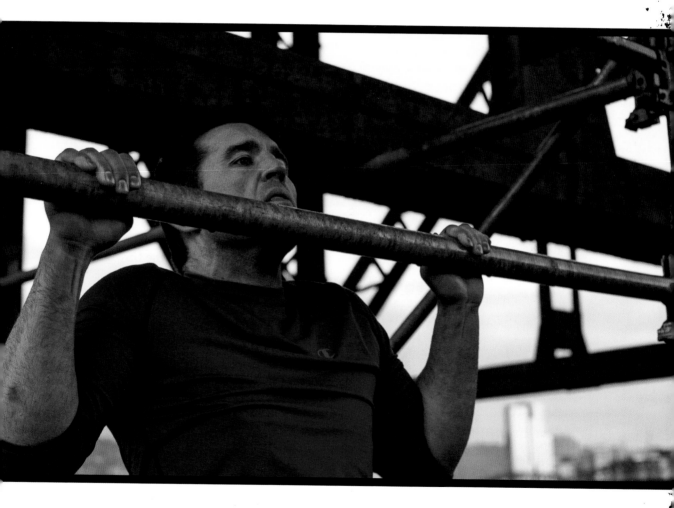

this—"Hey, we've got fettuccine incoming!"—and secrete insulin into the bloodstream to escort blood sugar (aka glucose) into all the cells in your body except the brain, which does not require any help from insulin. If there is more blood sugar than your cells can hold, insulin delivers the sugar to fat cells, where it is converted to and stored as fat. Insulin prevents high sugar levels in the blood, which can have some pretty damaging effects such as heart attack, stroke, and kidney and nerve damage. This is why, when some diabetics are alerted that their blood sugar levels are high, they inject insulin. This insulin escorts the excess sugar into the body's cells, keeping blood sugar levels in a safe range.

## What Causes Insulin Resistance?

Similar to leptin, it's possible to become resistant to insulin through poor dietary and lifestyle habits. Are you seeing a trend here? Processed carbs and sugar, inflammatory foods, and a lack of exercise are a few themes that will keep coming up over and over in this book.

Chronic, elevated blood sugar causes the pancreas to compensate by pumping out even more insulin in an attempt to reduce blood sugar. Over time, this excess insulin—a state called hyperinsulinemia—makes your cells more resistant as your blood becomes saturated with insulin and sugar. This can go on for only so long before the pancreas becomes damaged and your blood sugar skyrockets.

When our cells stop responding to insulin, a number of significant diseases can develop, including diabetes. Insulin resistance has become such a problem for modern humans that a study from 15 years ago showed that one-third of the US population may be insulin resistant. There are significant consequences that come with this, including heart disease, liver disease, Alzheimer's, and cancer. If you are wondering whether you have become resistant to insulin, your appearance and the food you eat will give you all the clues you need. Blood tests that check your level of triglycerides—the main form of fat in your bloodstream and stored in your body, covering those glorious abs—cholesterol, blood sugar, and insulin can give you an even clearer picture.

## How to Improve Insulin Sensitivity

Insulin resistance causes thousands of unnecessary deaths and instances of disease each year. Thankfully, you don't have to be one of these victims. Insulin is easy to influence, and resistance can often be reversed with changes to your diet and lifestyle–if you're willing to step up and do the work. Everything you need to do is explained in this book. We'll keep repeating our mantra: Move your body, eat healthy, manage stress, adapt, get some sleep, and enjoy spending time with the people you love. Not a bad way to live, right?

## STRATEGIES FOR HORMONE MANAGEMENT

As complicated as hormones are, managing them on a day-to-day basis is quite simple. Like driving a car, once you know how to turn it on and make it stop and go, you can travel from point A to point B with little conscious thought. Here are five actions you can take to get your hormones back on the right track. Start today and you will make an immediate difference in how your body functions.

### Eat Slow-Digesting Carbs

Carbs don't have to be the enemy. Ones that require extra time to digest are quite healthy. Legumes fit this profile. They are inexpensive, easy to prepare, and will immediately have a positive effective on hormone balance. (For more recipes and meal ideas, check out Chapter 9.)

### Avoid Sugar and Processed Carbohydrates

Gatorade, soda, sweetened cereals, candy, fruit juices–all that stuff. It's very easy to drink excessive amounts of sugar, so develop the habit of reading nutritional labels. You'll be surprised how much sugar many healthy-looking beverages contain. Let's include a few other carbs here as well, such as rice, potatoes, and pasta. It will take a few weeks of getting used to going without these items, but when your hormones begin to balance out, both your cravings for and enjoyment of these foods will reduce. Over time, with a reduction in weight and improvement in hormone fuction, when you do consume them, you'll be better equipped to process them.

### Focus on Whole Foods

Eating whole, natural foods including fatty fish, lean protein, nuts, and veggies will improve hormone sensitivity. In addition, stay away from processed meats and make a

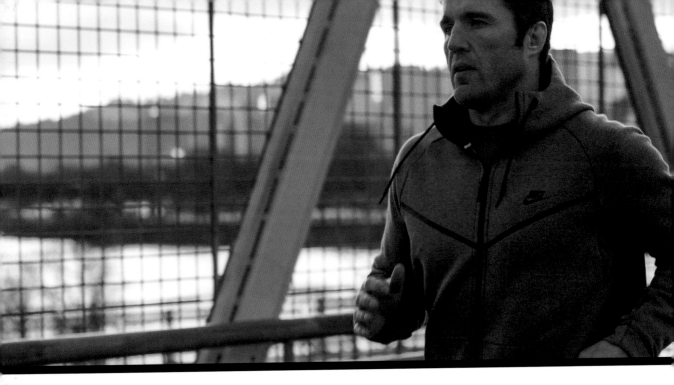

habit of reading nutrition labels. If what you're eating has six or more ingredients, odds are it's too processed to be healthy.

## Consume Omega-3 Fatty Acids (Essential Fats)

Essential fats are powerful compounds that reduce insulin resistance and lower triglycerides. They have profound effects on blood pressure regulation, liver function, the immune system, and your inflammatory response. Essential fats are necessary for the development of the brain and nervous system, hormone production, and proper thyroid and adrenal activity. Flax, hemp, and chia seeds are all excellent sources, along with fatty fish such as wild salmon. While we don't advocate a lot in the way of supplementation, fish oil is one supplement that can be beneficial to your diet.

## Resistance Training

The effect of exercise on insulin sensitivity is profound. It may be the simplest and easiest strategy for hormone optimization, and the effect is almost immediate. You may be surprised by how a small amount of exercise can make a difference. Scientists confirmed years ago that a single workout can increase the amount of glucose that insulin can escort into your cells for at least 16 hours afterward—and this was true even for people who did not previously exercise. In Chapter 6, we will let you in on a 10-minute workout that has been shown to give the benefits of 40 minutes of moderately paced cardio activity. And only 1 minute of those 10 is hard.

## SYSTEM RESET

So what happens to hormones with a weekly System Reset meal? Well, let's talk about leptin—the hormone produced in your fat cells that helps regulate body weight and appetite. When you start to lose weight, the level of leptin circulating in your body decreases, leading your brain to think you may be at risk of starvation. This can trigger your metabolism to slow down as your body conserves energy in order to survive. Just the opposite of what you want. This is where a System Reset meal may benefit you. One calorie-rich meal increases leptin levels long enough for your brain to recognize that all is good, and that there's no need to store excess fat. One caveat—you have to earn this meal. Eat well all week, work out, sleep, and manage stress. Once a week is beneficial; once a day is a killer.

## EVERYTHING YOU NEED TO KNOW

When too many hormones are secreted for extended periods of time, they lose their effectiveness. Eventually, these beneficial compounds end up doing us harm. As our body loses the ability to receive the valuable messages they deliver, it becomes easier to overeat, gain weight, feel stressed, and become sick.

Cortisol and adrenaline are masters at preparing our bodies to deal with any stressful situation. But as specialists, they are only needed for a few specific scenarios. The rest of the time these hormones should quiet down as you go about your business.

Insulin and leptin directly influence our appetite and how much of our food gets converted into fat. Severe health penalties are dished out when these hormones are unable to be utilized by our cells.

Thankfully, the best "medicine" for optimizing hormones does not need a prescription. At your next meal you can start to turn things around, and after just one workout your body will improve its ability to use these hormones as they were designed. So what are you waiting for?

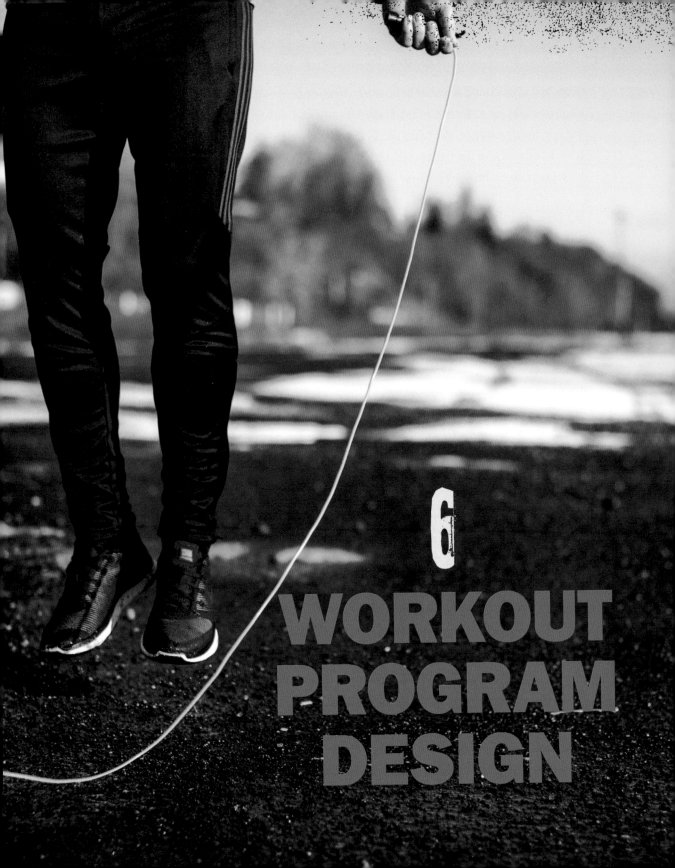

# 6
# WORKOUT PROGRAM DESIGN

**M**Y FATHER WAS A HORSEMAN, BREEDER OF THE YEAR A NUMBER OF TIMES. One day he got a call from a trainer named Tex Irwin, who said,. "Hey, there's a horse running on Saturday named Sun Vest; you need to buy this horse." And my dad said, "Why is that?" "Only I know how to train this horse," said Tex. "I know the secret to Sun Vest." So my dad picks up the horse and sure enough, Sun Vest wins five straight races—a track record. After his fifth win, he was sold for a handsome profit. But Sun Vest never won again.

Tex Irwin had figured out the secret to Sun Vest. Only he knew this particular horse did not like to work out hard and needed a different approach. If you wanted him to compete at his best, all he needed was to walk around the track once or twice. Never run him hard. On race day, he knew where that finish line was. And he really did: During the second of his five straight wins, there was a photo finish, and you could see him sticking his nose across the line to make sure he got there first. Sun Vest knew how to show up on game day. His best came from moderate effort. If you ran him hard every day, he wouldn't run fast on Saturday. Successful trainers customize training for each client based on their specific needs. It's not always possible, but any time you can make that happen, all the better. Find what works for you.

## PROGRAM DESIGN

Dr. Andy Galpin is a good friend of ours who runs the Center for Sport Performance at Cal State Fullerton, a leading exercise science lab contributing to the latest research in the field of human performance. He is unique because in addition to being a professor and a researcher, he was also a competitive Olympic weightlifter and coach. He understands fitness and performance from three unique vantage points—athlete, coach, and scientist.

One of the classes he teaches is called Program Design. As a final project, students are required to write a yearlong workout program for a client—it could be their mother, a professional athlete, or anyone in between. Let's pretend for a moment that you are a student in Dr. Galpin's class. You must consider your client's goals, lifestyle, and current fitness level when creating their workout program. Their unique genetic strengths and limitations, personality, motivation, economic status, and work schedule, as well as potential pitfalls, must be accounted for. As you know, even with the best intentions, planning, and support, we all get pushed off course from time to time. Holidays, vacations, sickness–sometimes we just need a break. For students to receive a passing grade from Dr. Galpin, each program must account for all areas of the client's life. In our opinion, these considerations are the foundation of lasting change.

There is no one "perfect" workout. Even if you found one that you thought fit the bill, your body would eventually adapt to the exercises and your progress would slow. This is an efficiency mechanism designed to conserve energy. Remember, your body still thinks it's living in caveman times. To maximize the effects of each workout, strength and conditioning specialists use a strategy called periodization, in which the same workout is never repeated for very long. While it may seem like a fancy concept, it's really not. It's just about doing things in cycles. Just as day turns into night and winter transforms into spring, we shift our training from short-term goals to long-term lifestyle maintenance and back again. Change is always occurring, and adaptation is how you create and maintain success. Master these cycles and you will master your life.

When thinking about your approach to a four-pack, imagine you are a student of Dr. Galpin's. Look at yourself in the same way he asks his students to consider their client's needs. On a piece of paper, write down the variables and challenges in your own life and consider how you're going to accommodate them. This way, when challenges do arise, you'll have a game plan to follow and won't be thrown off course. A four-pack is great, but a solid four-pack is even better. This is achieved by building muscle, and the only way to build calorie-burning, lean muscle is through resistance exercise. Keep in mind that there's a limit to the amount of calories you can burn by working out. If your diet is not dialed in for fat loss and you are eating excess calories, especially from the wrong sources, then all the cardio in the world won't help you reach your goals. This is why we rely on food to reduce body fat. ("Abs are made in the kitchen" is a saying bodybuilders have been using for as long as there have been bodybuilders.) The type of training program you need combines both strength training and cardiovascular exercise. The good news is that no matter what equipment you have available—from your living room to a membership at a fully equipped gym—you can build muscle, burn fat, and sculpt the four-pack of your dreams.

If you haven't been working out consistently, a regular exercise routine will be a change to your lifestyle. But you may be surprised by how little time you need to invest to see results. Consider the best time and place for your workouts and what resources you'll need to be successful. This may mean a gym membership, a new pair of hiking boots, a workout buddy, or a personal trainer.

Plan workouts that fit your schedule and personal preferences. I prefer to work out mid-morning. For Ryan, late afternoon is best. If you have limited time, go for short, high-intensity circuits. These burn calories including fat, while strengthening your heart and building lean muscle. Lastly, we are not relying on exercise to lose weight; we are building lean muscle to keep our metabolism and hormones functioning optimally. Four-Pack foods will take care of the rest.

## Fat-Burning Zone

Most of us spend more time thinking about losing fat than we do about gaining muscle. Luckily for us, the body is designed to burn fat—it just needs the right environment to do so. There are a few myths when it comes to burning fat and losing weight. The most mis-understood is the "fat-burning zone."

Your body burns a combination of carbohydrates and fat; it's almost never just one or the other. At 50 percent of your maximum heart rate, you will be burning fuel at a ratio of 60 percent fat and 40 percent carbohydrates, in the form of glycogen that is stored in the body. When you increase to 75 percent of your maximum heart rate, the ratio drops to 35 percent fat and 65 percent carbs. Therefore, it may seem logical that workouts done at a lower heart rate would make the most sense for those looking to shed a few pounds. But in reality, you burn more total calories by working harder. So even though the ratio of fat-to-carbs is lower at higher intensities, more total fat and calories are expended.

New research is published every year demonstrating the benefits of intense exercise. Magic happens when you get your heart rate up and feel your chest pounding. Short, intense interval training workouts are beneficial because much of the physiological benefits of exercise come when you really push the pace, even if it's only for a minute or two. If you don't have access to gym equipment or are short on time, then a high-intensity interval training (HIIT) workout with body-weight exercises such as squats, burpees, and jumping jacks can still deliver amazing results, all in the comfort of your own home. No gym membership, no weights, no excuses.

## Why It Pays to Train Hard

The benefits of exercise are no secret. But besides the obvious advantage of building muscle and burning fat, regular exercise will pay dividends in others areas of your life as well. Here are 10 benefits to exercise.

1.  **You'll sleep better.** There's solid, scientific evidence linking regular exercise with improved sleep patterns. Just 20 to 30 minutes a day, three or four times a week will do the job. Falling asleep becomes easier, and you'll spend more time in the deepest stages of sleep. If you are someone who prefers to work out at night, make sure it's not too close to bedtime. You may find yourself lying in bed, wired and unable to keep still.

2.  **You'll age better.** Do you know what one of the most significant indicators of longevity is? Leg strength. Not being able to go to the bathroom unassisted is one reason why many people end up in assisted living facilities. There have been a number of studies that have demonstrated the value of strong muscles, especially leg strength. In 2008, a study from the Unit for Preventive Nutrition at Karolinska Institute in Sweden linked increased muscle strength to a lower risk of death and cancer. In 2010 and 2012, the Feinberg School of Medicine at Northwestern University in Chicago published studies that found in men with peripheral arterial disease, the weaker their leg strength was, the more likely they were to die. It pays to be strong–not just mentally, but physically. Strong legs enable you to move easier. This increases your ability to remain physically active as you age, keeping your heart healthy. Strong muscles also improve balance while reducing your risk of falling. The University of Maryland Medical School

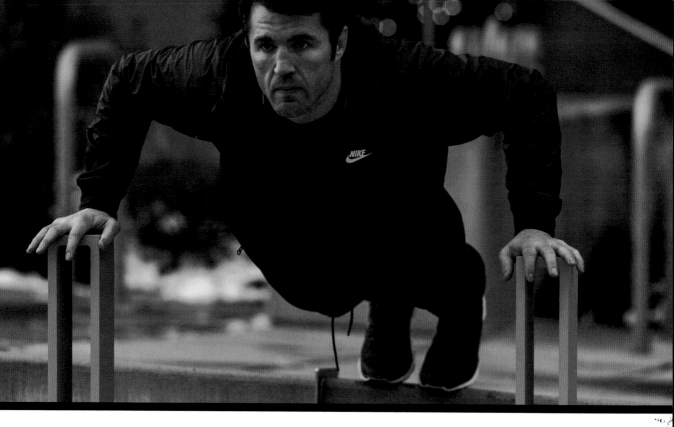

published a study in 2006 that stated 29 percent of people who break their hips from falls die within a year. All the more reason to making building muscle a priority. As we age, there's a natural decrease in aerobic capacity and muscle mass, but you can reverse or slow this process with exercise. In addition, the risk of many age-related diseases such as osteoporosis, stroke, and heart disease decreases with exercise.

3. **You'll be stronger, more flexible, and athletic.** Healthy bones, muscles, and joints are needed at every stage in life. Even a moderate exercise program will deliver these benefits.

4. **Your immune system will be more effective.** Exercise is a powerful way to stimulate the production of natural immune cells, and a stronger body is better equipped to fight off infectious diseases. This is an added benefit to strength training that many people do not consider.

5. **You'll become mentally sharper.** If better memory, reaction time, and concentration are skills you think are valuable, then you're in luck. Harvard Medical School researchers have found a powerful molecule called irisin that the body releases after moderate aerobic activity. Irisin helps maintain healthy body weight, improves cognition, and may even slow the aging process. It doesn't require much effort to get these benefits either: Light cardio three or four times a week will do the job.

6. **You'll become more confident.** Confidence is a trait many people lack. Feeling good about yourself and having the courage to go after what you want in life is a gift not only for you but also for those around you. It can be hard to be confident when you are overweight. Step up, do the work, and earn the rewards. You will start to feel the difference physically and mentally within a few weeks.

7. **You'll have more energy.** It may seem counterintuitive, but the more energy you spend, the more you will have. We all have those days when we are too tired to work out. But there have been times when you made the effort anyway and felt energized afterward. You are not destined to feel slow and tired for the rest of your life.

8. **You'll be better in bed.** No, really. When you work out more, you'll develop a stronger sex drive and will do the deed better and with more satisfaction. Increased strength and endurance will pay off in the long run as well. Exercise decreases your chance of erectile dysfunction, especially as you age. If this alone doesn't motivate you, we're not sure what else to say.

9. **You'll reduce stress, anxiety, and depression.** We all hold tension, stress, and emotions in our muscles, and exercise depletes this energy in an empowering way. The release of your brain's feel-good neurotransmitters, called endorphins, following exercise will boost your mood and promote relaxation. It will also help provide motivation to eat better. If you are prone to depression, working out may be the single best thing you can do for yourself, and there is a lot of research behind this recommendation. The bigger problem was highlighted in the academic journal *Sports Medicine* in 2014, in which a paper was published that examined 168 studies on how stress impacts physical activity. Not surprisingly, the studies revealed that when people experience stress, they find being active

much more difficult—all the more reason to form good habits, surround yourself with healthy, like-minded people, and have a plan for when stress levels rise and motivation decreases. Your physical and mental health depend on it.

10. **You'll look better.** Vanity is not dead! Sometimes it's better to look good than to feel good. Fortunately, with the Four-Pack plan, you do not have to choose one over the other.

## Have It Your Way

We have stressed throughout this book the importance of creating a plan that fits you. If you don't find food you enjoy eating and exercise that is fun to do, how can you possibly expect to sustain this behavior over the long haul? It may not be conscious, but your natural tendencies will eventually take over and you'll find a way to reject your new plan before too long. A version of this happens in mixed martial arts fights all the time. When fighters find themselves in trouble, they often revert back to their original style of martial arts. For example, a wrestler will keep trying to shoot takedowns even if they're not successful with the technique. Stress exposes our patterns and highlights our weaknesses. If a Big Mac represents comfort, chances are you will find yourself at the McDonald's drive-thru when you become stressed. It's possible to break these unhealthy habits, but it requires self-awareness and discipline.

John Parsons (Ryan's father) was a former All-American wrestler. At an age when most people retire, he exchanged the wrestling shoes of his youth for hiking boots and trekked the entire length of the 2,200-mile Appalachian Trail—twice. This historic hike begins at Springer Mountain in Georgia and traverses through 14 states before ending at the summit of Mount Katahdin in Maine. Since John works full-time, he broke the hike up into sections and completed them over several years. It wasn't uncommon for him to cover as many as 720 miles and lose 30 pounds during one of his 6-week hikes on the trail. Hiking upward of 20 miles a day from morning to night burns a lot of calories. Eating high-calorie foods such as peanut butter helped sustain him, but given the ground he was covering, it was inevitable that his body would turn to itself for much-needed calories. There's another lesson here: John did this in his late sixties and now, at 70, he's still at it. This goes to show that it's never too late. Your body will respond to exercise at any age.

Now, as impressive as this is, John experienced what many long-distance athletes do after returning home: He continued to eat like he was still hiking 12 hours a day. Those 30 pounds that melted away while walking through the woods came back with a vengeance. Following one of his lengthy hiking excursions, it was not uncommon for John to find himself at Starbucks getting his morning coffee—and ordering three muffins to go with it. It took conscious effort to remember that he didn't need 10,000 calories a day to survive. Remember, your body isn't aware of the bigger picture, so you need to be in charge, steering the ship.

There are many different ways to exercise. From a yoga class to hitting a heavy bag, a walk around the block to an intense CrossFit workout—there is no one-size-fits-all approach. So experiment and find activities that you enjoy. Better yet, find several options to keep things interesting and your body guessing. If you're looking for a place to start, keep reading.

## FOUR-PACK WARMUPS

What gets ignored more: warming up or stretching? It's a toss-up. Like stretching, there are a lot of benefits that come with taking a few minutes to get your body primed for action. Along with improving range of motion and reducing the risk of injury, a warmup provides time to get mentally ready to work out. If you train with friends, it's also a fun time to connect socially.

## CORE CARDIO WORKOUTS

Life is hectic, and a daily workout is easy to bump off the priority list. That excuse is now over—meet the 10-Minute Core Cardio workout. There are a number of variations, which are easy to customize to meet your specific needs. If you don't have a stationary bike, a pair of running shoes or simple body-weight exercises requiring no equipment will do just fine. We love these workouts because you can always find 10 minutes in your day to fit one in.

Variations of short, intense workouts have been used for years in mixed martial arts, but in 2016 researchers at McMaster University in Canada claimed that sprinting for three 20-second intervals, spread out over 10 minutes, was equal to 45 minutes of moderate cardio. This seemed too good to be true, so Ryan headed up to Dr. Galpin's lab and they ran some tests. What they learned is that yes, this is possible. But during each sprint interval, you must push as hard as you possibly can; maximum effort is required if you want to

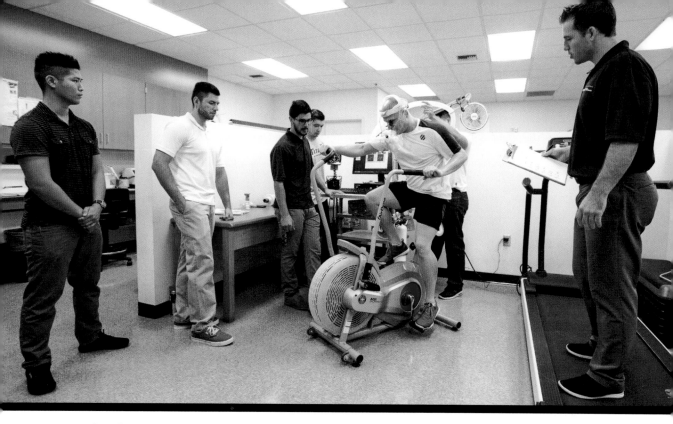

Ryan Parsons testing the Four-Pack workouts with Dr. Andy Galpin.

reap the maximum benefit. There's still value in the workout if you don't give your max intensity, though, as sprinting for any amount of time delivers additional benefits.

Included are four variations of the 10-Minute Core Cardio Workout. The difference between each is the number of sprints performed. As you progress, you'll add more sprints in the same amount of time. It is very simple to modify these workouts with any type of cardio equipment, or even an inexpensive rebound trampoline. The key is to give maximum effort at whatever you are doing for 20 seconds, followed by light movement

## FOUR-PACK WARMUP

| GENERAL PREP X 2 | REPS |
|---|---|
| Jumping Jacks | 15 |
| Seal Jacks | 15 |
| Squats/Sumo Squats | 10 |
| Pushups/Yoga Pushups | 10 |

## CORE CARDIO 1

**EQUIPMENT NEEDED:** Stationary bike

**TIME:** 10 minutes

**NOTES:** Variations of this workout can be done on a treadmill, elliptical, rower, VersaClimber, stairs, rebound trampoline, and the road or field.

| LEVEL 1 | PACE | |
| --- | --- | --- |
| Minute 1 | easy | |
| Minute 2 | moderate | |
| Minute 3 | moderate | |
| Minute 4 | **20 sec sprint** | *40 sec moderate* |
| Minute 5 | moderate | |
| Minute 6 | **20 sec sprint** | *40 sec moderate* |
| Minute 7 | moderate | |
| Minute 8 | **20 sec sprint** | *40 sec moderate* |
| Minute 9 | moderate | |
| Minute 10 | moderate | |

## CORE CARDIO 2

| LEVEL 1 | PACE | |
| --- | --- | --- |
| Minute 1 | easy | |
| Minute 2 | moderate | |
| Minute 3 | **20 sec sprint** | *40 sec moderate* |
| Minute 4 | moderate | |
| Minute 5 | **20 sec sprint** | *40 sec moderate* |
| Minute 6 | moderate | |
| Minute 7 | **20 sec sprint** | *40 sec moderate* |
| Minute 8 | moderate | |
| Minute 9 | **20 sec sprint** | *40 sec moderate* |
| Minute 10 | moderate | |

## CORE CARDIO 3

| LEVEL 1 | | PACE |
|---|---|---|
| Minute 1 | easy | |
| Minute 2 | **20 sec sprint** | *40 sec moderate* |
| Minute 3 | moderate | |
| Minute 4 | **20 sec sprint** | *40 sec moderate* |
| Minute 5 | **20 sec sprint** | *40 sec moderate* |
| Minute 6 | moderate | |
| Minute 7 | **20 sec sprint** | *40 sec moderate* |
| Minute 8 | **20 sec sprint** | *40 sec moderate* |
| Minute 9 | moderate | |
| Minute 10 | moderate | |

## CORE CARDIO 4

| LEVEL 1 | | PACE |
|---|---|---|
| Minute 1 | easy | |
| Minute 2 | **20 sec sprint** | *40 sec moderate* |
| Minute 3 | **20 sec sprint** | *40 sec moderate* |
| Minute 4 | **20 sec sprint** | *40 sec moderate* |
| Minute 5 | **20 sec sprint** | *40 sec moderate* |
| Minute 6 | **20 sec sprint** | *40 sec moderate* |
| Minute 7 | **20 sec sprint** | *40 sec moderate* |
| Minute 8 | **20 sec sprint** | *40 sec moderate* |
| Minute 9 | **20 sec sprint** | *40 sec moderate* |
| Minute 10 | moderate | |

# HIGH-INTENSITY INTERVAL WORKOUTS

## WORKOUT 1: STRENGTH & METABOLIC

**EQUIPMENT NEEDED:** 2 dumbbells or kettlebells, stability ball

**ESTIMATED DURATION:** 40 mins—2 rounds, 60 min—3 rounds

**NOTES:** Perform exercises as a circuit following the prescribed work and rest times.

| EXERCISE | WORK | REST |
|---|---|---|
| 1. DB Squat | 60 sec | 30 sec |
| 2. Squat Jumps | 30 sec | 30 sec |
| 3. Pushups | 60 sec | 30 sec |
| 4. Mountain Climbers | 30 sec | 30 sec |
| 5. Stability Ball Glute Bridge | 60 sec | 30 sec |
| 6. Kettlebell Swings | 30 sec | 30 sec |

*Rest 30 seconds and repeat x 2-3 rounds*

| REST 2 MINUTES BETWEEN CIRCUITS | | |
|---|---|---|
| 1. DB Bent-Over Row | 60 sec | 30 sec |
| 2. Medicine Ball Slam | 30 sec | 30 sec |
| 3. Alternating Lateral Lunge | 60 sec | 30 sec |
| 4. Skater Hops | 30 sec | 30 sec |
| 5. DB Curl & Press | 60 sec | 30 sec |
| 6. Stability Ball Stir the Pot | 30 sec | 30 sec |

*Rest 20 seconds and repeat x 2-3 rounds*

# DB SQUAT

1. Stand up straight while holding a dumbbell in each hand (palms facing the sides of your legs).

2. Position your feet in a shoulder-width stance with the toes slightly pointed out. Keep your head up at all times, as looking down can put you off balance, and also maintain a straight back. This will be your starting position.

3. Slowly lower your torso by bending your knees and sending your butt backward, as you maintain a straight back and keep your head up. Continue down until your thighs are parallel to the floor.

4. Raise your torso by pushing the floor away through the heels of your feet as you straighten the legs and return to the starting position.

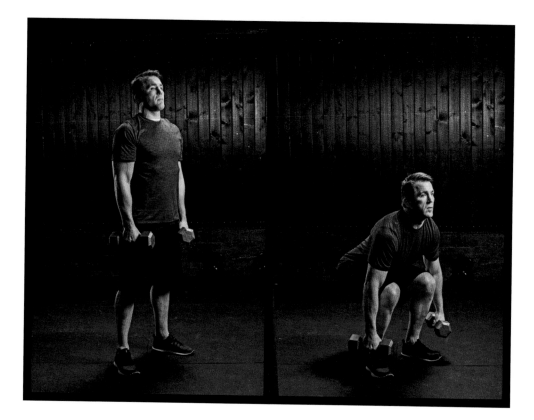

# SQUAT JUMPS

1. Stand with your feet shoulder-width apart.

2. Start by doing a regular squat, then engage your core and jump up explosively.

3. When you land, lower your body back into the squat position to complete one rep. Land as softly and in control as possible.

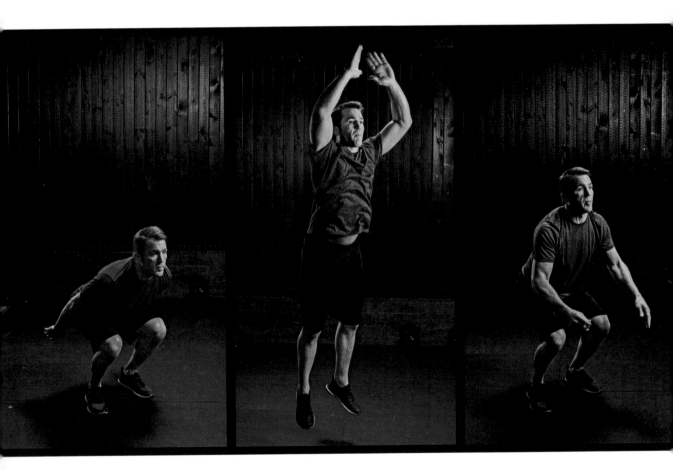

# PUSHUPS

1. Get into plank position, with your hands under but slightly outside of your shoulders.

2. Lower your body until your chest touches or nearly touches the floor. As you lower, keep your elbows tucked into your sides, pulling them close to your body so your upper arms form a 45-degree angle when your torso is in the bottom position of the move.

3. Pause at the bottom, then push back to the starting position. Keep your core braced the entire time and do not let your hips sag at any point during the exercise.

4. If placing your hands directly on the floor hurts your wrists, find a pair of dumbbells with flat surfaces (like hex dumbbells) and place them where you would position your hands. Grasp the dumbbells' handles and keep your wrists straight as you perform the exercise.

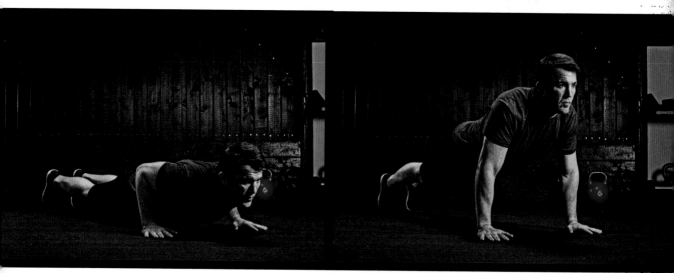

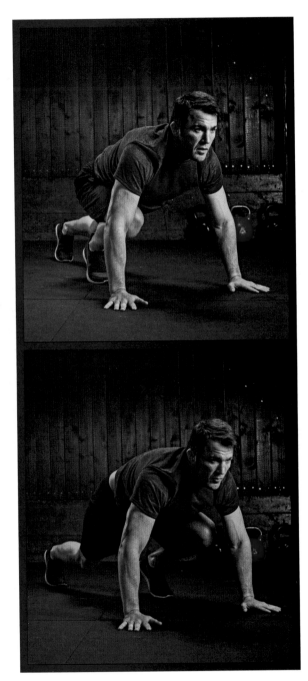

## MOUNTAIN CLIMBERS

1. Begin in a pushup plank position, with your weight supported by your hands and toes.

2. Bend your right knee and hip, bringing your leg under you until your knee is approximately under your right hip (think of a sprinter start position). This will be your starting position.

3. Explosively reverse the positions of your legs, extending the right leg until it is straight and supported by the toe and lifting the left foot and bringing the left knee toward the left hip.

4. Repeat in an alternating fashion for 20 to 30 seconds.

# STABILITY BALL
# GLUTE BRIDGE

1.  Rest your head and shoulders on the floor with your knees bent at a 90-degree angle and heels resting on a stability ball.

2.  Make sure that your knees are stacked over your ankles.

3.  Keep your arms folded behind your head or against the floor and press the hips toward the ceiling. Don't let your thighs and butt sink back toward the ground. Keep everything tight and pressed upward.

4.  Slowly lower your hips down to starting position.

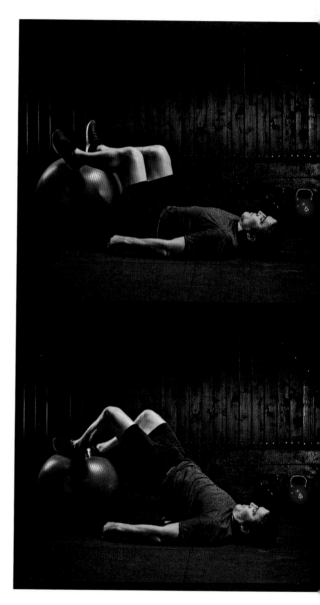

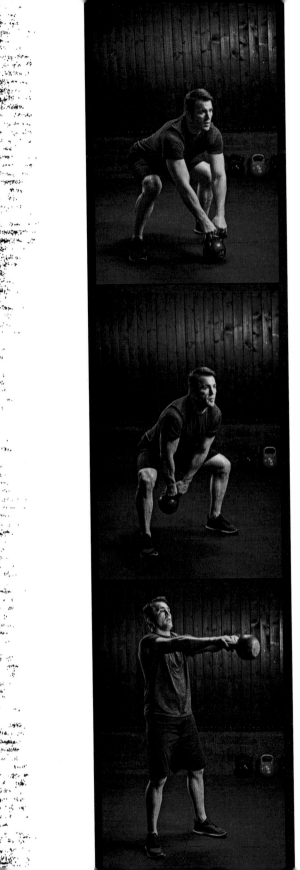

## KETTLEBELL SWINGS

1. Stand over the kettlebell with feet shoulder width apart, chest up, and shoulders back and down. The kettlebell should be about 8 to 12 inches in front of your feet, forming a triangle with your two feet and the kettlebell.

2. Send your hips backward, keeping your body weight in your heels. Reach down with long and loose arms and grip the kettlebell with your palms facing you and thumbs wrapped loosely around the handle. Keep your shoulder blades back and down and tighten your core.

3. Once you have tension throughout your body, hike the kettlebell back between your legs.

4. Driving through your heels, explode through the hips to send the weight swinging upward by tensing your glutes, keeping your core tight, and generating power from your hips. Aim for chest height, keeping the arms extended.

5. As the kettlebell begins to descend, let the weight do the work as you ready your body for the next rep. Shift your weight back into your heels while hinging at the hips and loading both the hamstrings and glutes. Receive the weight by allowing the kettlebell to swing back between the legs.

# DB BENT-OVER ROW

1. With a dumbbell in each hand (palms facing your torso), bend your knees slightly and bend forward at the waist. As you bend, make sure to keep your back straight. Bend forward until your back is almost parallel to the floor.

2. While keeping your torso stationary, lift the dumbbells to your side as you breathe out, keeping the elbows close to the body. Do not curl the dumbbells or exert any force with the forearm other than holding the weights.

3. At the top of the row, squeeze your back muscles and hold for a second.

4. Slowly lower the weight again to the starting position as you inhale.

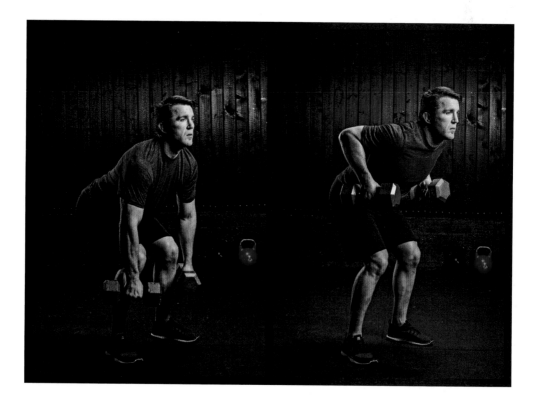

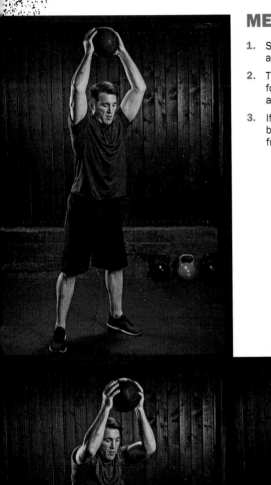

## MEDICINE BALL SLAM

1. Stand with your feet shoulder width apart and knees slightly bent, and hold a non-bouncing medicine ball overhead.

2. Throw the ball down to the ground in front of your feet with as much force as possible. Exhale during the movement and contract your abs.

3. If possible, catch the ball as it bounces from the floor. If there's no bounce at all, keep the ab muscles engaged and pick the ball up from the floor.

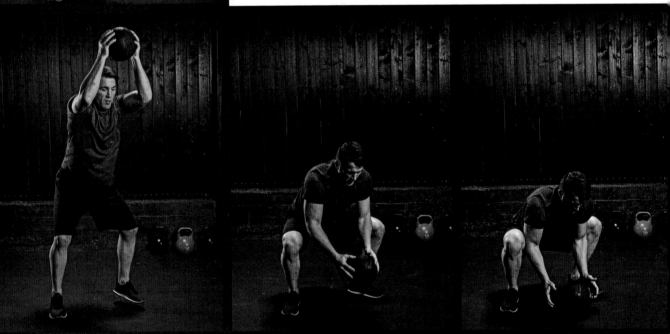

# ALTERNATING LATERAL LUNGE

1. From standing, step far out to the right with your right leg.

2. Bend your right knee and sit back to lower into a side lunge, keeping your back flat and chest up.

3. Press through the right foot to return to your start position and then repeat on your left leg.

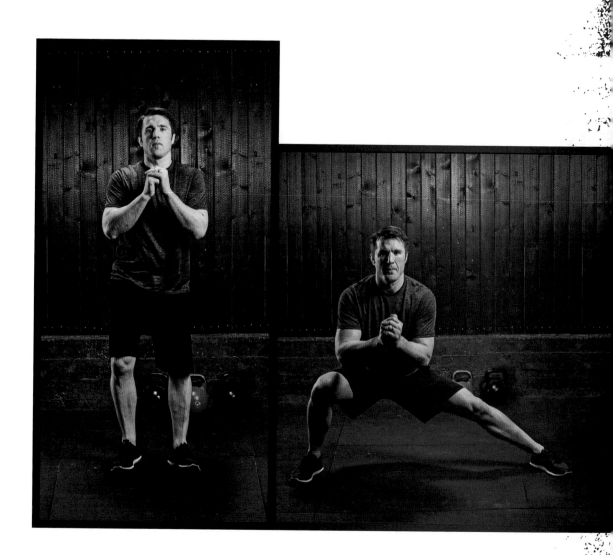

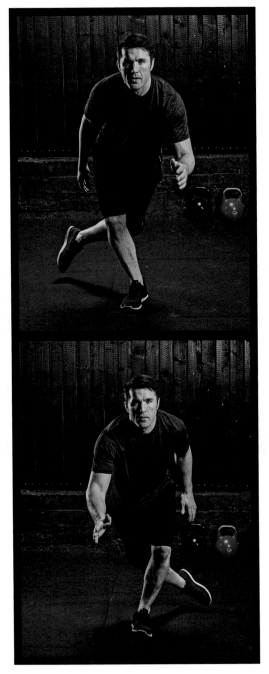

## SKATER HOPS

1. Stand on your right foot with your right knee slightly bent and your left foot slightly off the floor.

2. Dip your knees and lower your body toward the floor, then bound to your left by jumping off your right foot.

3. Land on your left foot and at the same time allow your right foot to travel behind you and your right arm to cross in front of you.

4. Reverse the movement, landing on your right foot.

# DB CURL & PRESS

1. Begin in a standing position with your feet shoulder width apart and a dumbbell in each hand. Your arms should be hanging at your sides. Look directly ahead, keeping your chest up.

2. Initiate the movement by flexing the elbows to curl the weight to your shoulders. Do not use momentum or flex through the shoulder. Use a controlled motion.

3. Execute the pressing movement by extending your arms as you press the weight above your head. You should finish the press with your palms facing either inward or forward.

4. Pause at the top of the motion before reversing to return to the starting position.

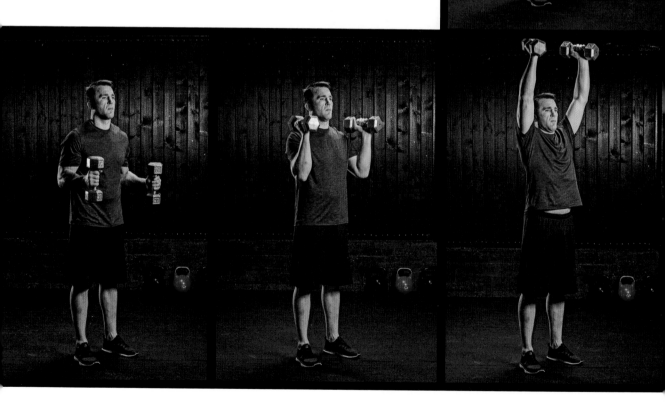

## STABILITY BALL STIR THE POT

1. Position a stability ball in front of you and rest your knees on a mat.

2. Place your forearms on the stability ball. While bracing through your core, raise your knees off the floor. You are performing a plank on the ball. Your ankles, hips, and shoulders should form a straight line. Do not let your hips sag.

3. Use your forearms to move the ball in small circles in a "stirring" motion.

4. Perform half of the recommended repetitions circling clockwise, then switch to perform the other half counterclockwise.

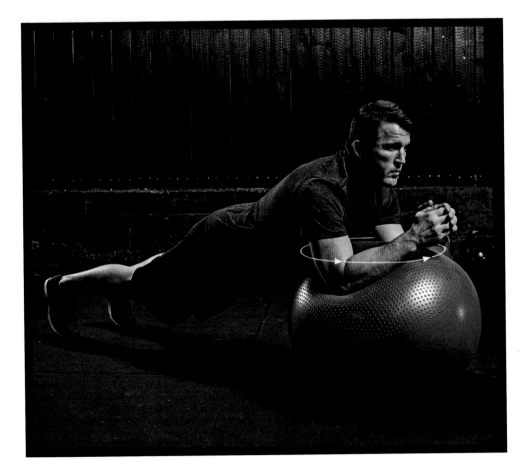

## WORKOUT 2: STRENGTH & METABOLIC

**EQUIPMENT NEEDED:** 2 dumbbells or kettlebells, stability ball, markers or cones

**ESTIMATED DURATION:** 40 mins—2 rounds, 60 min—3 rounds

**NOTES:** Perform exercises as a circuit following the prescribed work and rest times.

| EXERCISE | WORK | REST |
|---|---|---|
| 1. DB Reverse Lunge with Knee Drive | 60 sec | 30 sec |
| 2. High Knees | 30 sec | 30 sec |
| 3. Renegade Row | 60 sec | 30 sec |
| 4. Alternating Sit-Outs | 30 sec | 30 sec |
| 5. Squat Holds | 60 sec | 30 sec |
| 6. 5-Yard Repeat Shuffle | 30 sec | 30 sec |

*Rest 30 seconds and repeat x 2-3 rounds*

| REST 2 MINUTES BETWEEN CIRCUITS | | |
|---|---|---|
| 1. DB RDL | 60 sec | 30 sec |
| 2. Broad Jump | 30 sec | 30 sec |
| 3. Lunge Stance DB Overhead Press | 60 sec | 30 sec |
| 4. Jumping Jacks | 30 sec | 30 sec |
| 5. One-Arm Pushup Hold | 60 sec | 30 sec |
| 6. In & Out Hops | 30 sec | 30 sec |

*Rest 20 seconds and repeat x 2-3 rounds*

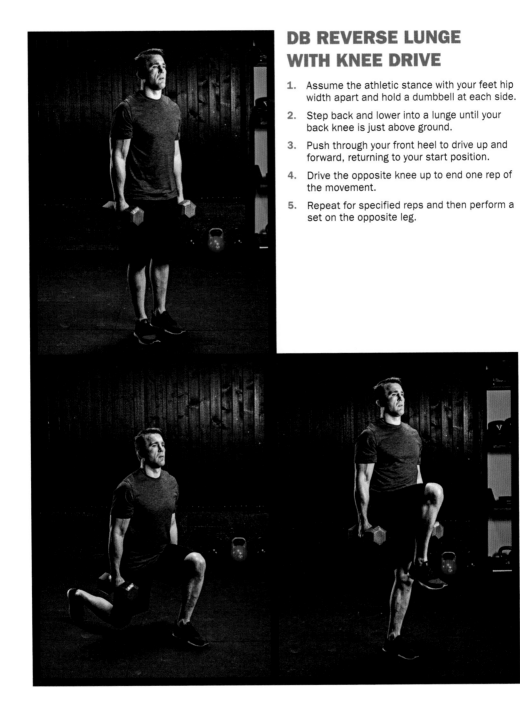

## DB REVERSE LUNGE WITH KNEE DRIVE

1. Assume the athletic stance with your feet hip width apart and hold a dumbbell at each side.

2. Step back and lower into a lunge until your back knee is just above ground.

3. Push through your front heel to drive up and forward, returning to your start position.

4. Drive the opposite knee up to end one rep of the movement.

5. Repeat for specified reps and then perform a set on the opposite leg.

# HIGH KNEES

1. Stand straight with the feet hip width apart. Look straight ahead and let your arms hang by your sides.

2. Jump from one foot to the other, lifting your knees as high as possible (like you are running in place). Hip height would be a great target height.

3. Your arms should follow the motion. Lift your right arm as your left knee comes up and vice versa.

4. Touch the ground with the balls of your feet only. Stay light and fast.

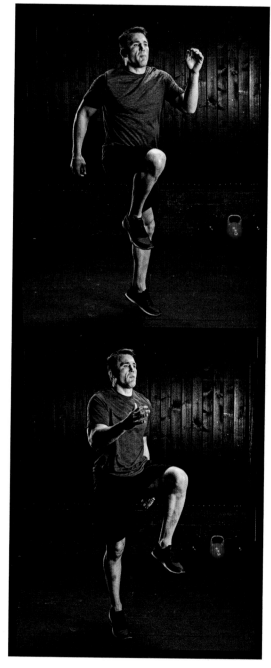

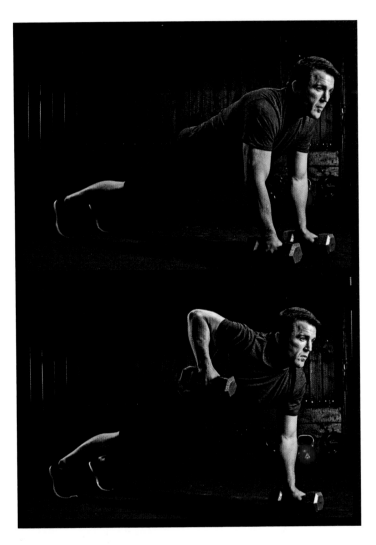

## RENEGADE ROW

1.  Place two dumbbells or kettlebells about shoulder width apart on the floor and assume a pushup position with your hands on the handles. Keep your core tight and do not let your hips sag throughout this exercise.

2.  Push hard into the ground with your left hand (keeping your elbow locked) while simultaneously pulling the weight to your waist with your right hand.

3.  Lower the weight back to the starting position under control.

4.  Repeat this motion, alternating the lifting arm.

# ALTERNATING SIT-OUTS

1. Get into a pushup plank position on your hands and toes.

2. Shift your weight to your left hand and step forward slightly with your right foot as you turn your body to the right.

3. Pull your right hand back to your right shoulder as you turn your body and kick your left leg through (perpendicular to your start position). Your weight will now all be on your left hand and right foot.

4. Return to the center and repeat on the opposite side.

5. Continue alternating sides.

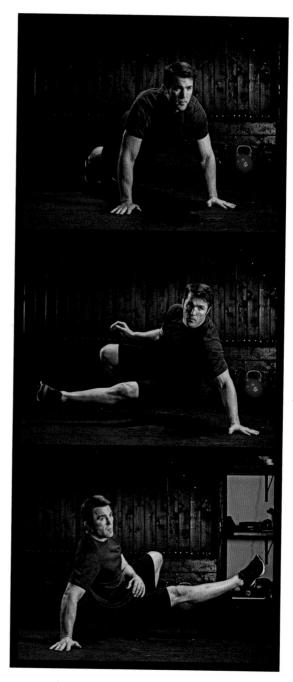

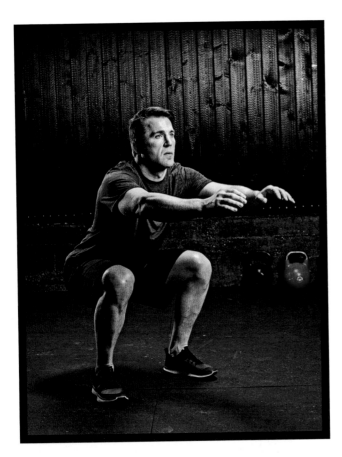

## SQUAT HOLDS

1. Start with feet slightly wider than hip width apart, toes slight pointing out.

2. Engage your core, and while keeping your back in a neutral position, slowly sit your hips back as though you are sitting into a chair. Don't let your knees cave inward—keep your knees tracking in line with your feet.

3. Only sit back as far as is comfortable. You shouldn't feel any pain in your knees or other joints. Advanced trainees should squat down to where their thighs are parallel to the ground and the bend in their knee forms a 90-degree angle. Intermediate trainees should aim for a 60-degree angle and beginners a 30-degree angle.

4. Actively engage the glutes by clenching your butt cheeks together. Concentrate on squeezing to hold yourself in the squat position.

5. Place your hands either on your hips or extended straight out in front of you.

6. Hold this position for up to 1 minute.

# 5-YARD REPEAT SHUFFLE

1. Start with 2 markers, lines, cones, etc., 5 yards apart. Face marker 1 in a 2-point athletic stance.

2. Push off your right foot taking short shuffle steps to the left until you hit the other marker.

3. Touch the marker with your left hand, then immediately push off your left foot and shuffle back to the start.

4. Continue to repeat this pattern, touching as many markers as you can in the allotted time.

5. Be sure to keep your knees bent, hips low, back flat, and chest up (athletic position) the whole time.

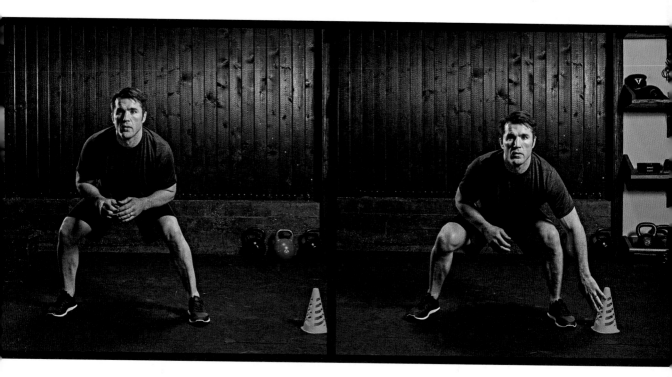

# DB RDL

1. Begin in a standing position with a dumbbell in each hand. Ensure that your back is straight and stays that way for the duration of the exercise. Allow your arms to hang perpendicular to the floor, with the palms facing your thighs and the elbows pointed out to your sides.

2. Flex your hips, slowly pushing your butt back. This should entail a horizontal movement of the hips, rather than a downward movement. The knees should only partially bend (the degree may vary depending on your flexibility) and your weight should remain on your heels.

3. Drive your butt back as far as you can. This should generate tension in your hamstrings as your hands approach knee level. Maintain an arch in your back throughout the exercise.

4. When your hips cannot perform any further backward movement, pause, and then slowly return to the starting position by extending your hips.

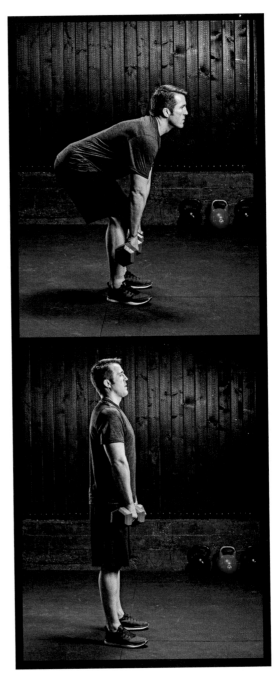

# BROAD JUMP

1. Stand up straight with feet about shoulder width apart.

2. Drop into a deep squat and swing both arms back.

3. Swing the arms forward and extend the knees and hips to jump forward.

4. Land on both feet and stand upright.

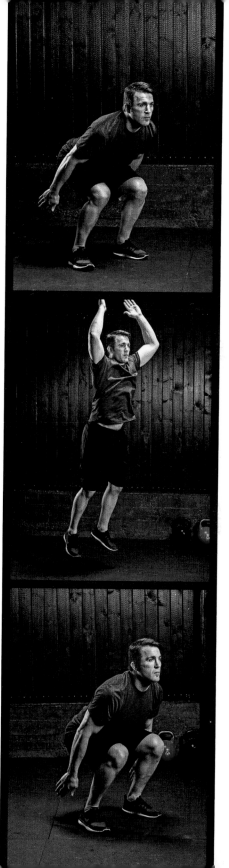

# LUNGE STANCE
# DB OVERHEAD PRESS

1. Stand with your feet about shoulder width apart, holding dumbbells by your sides.

2. Step your left leg forward into a lunge, being mindful that your left knee should wind up positioned above your ankle and not over your toes.

3. Maintaining the lunge position with your torso upright, curl the dumbbells to your shoulders, and then press the dumbbells overhead, finishing with your elbows straight and your biceps by your ears.

4. Lower the dumbbells to your shoulders, then press up again.

5. Perform half the reps (or time) with your left leg forward, then switch legs and continue until you complete the set.

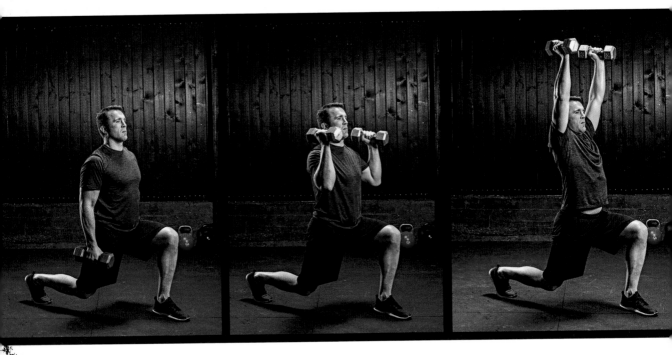

# JUMPING JACKS

1. Stand with your feet together and your hands by your sides, palms touching your thighs.

2. In one motion, jump your feet out to the side and raise your arms above your head.

3. Immediately reverse that motion by jumping back to the starting position, then repeat in a continuous sequence.

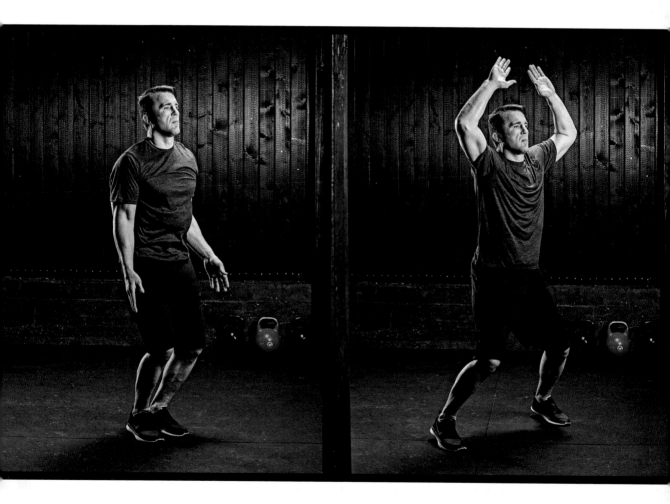

# ONE-ARM PUSHUP HOLD
# (SWITCH AS NEEDED)

1. Begin in the pushup plank position with hands 6 to 8 inches apart and fingers facing forward.

2. Spread your feet so they are slightly outside shoulder width apart.

3. Brace through your core like you were about to get kicked in the stomach, and squeeze your glutes.

4. Push down through your feet and your right hand, while lifting your left hand off the floor and gently touch your right shoulder.

5. Maintain a perfect straight body plank position, keeping your hips facing the floor and moving slowly and with control the whole time.

6. Pretend there is a cup of water on your low back and you can't allow it to spill during any movement.

7. When your arm begins to fatigue (or as you wish), switch hands slowly, not allowing anything else to move.

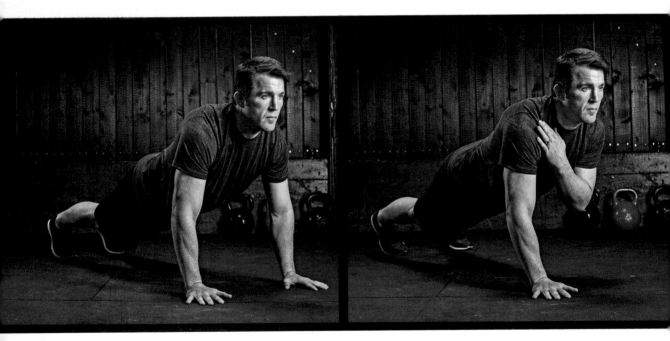

# IN & OUT HOPS

1.  Start in an athletic position with your knees bent, hips low, chest up, and feet shoulder width apart.

2.  Staying low, quickly hop until your feet are a few inches apart, then hop back to the start position.

3.  Repeat continuously as quickly as possible, staying low with only the balls of your feet touching the ground.

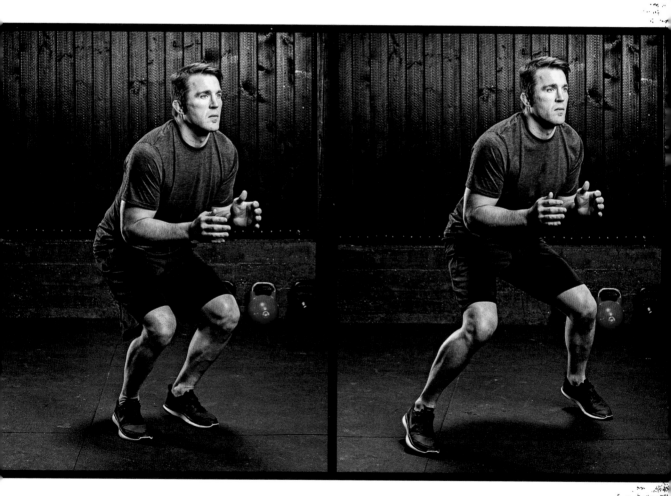

## WORKOUT 3: PYRAMID

**EQUIPMENT NEEDED:** 6-inch box or step, 2 weights (any type), jump rope, stability ball

**ESTIMATED DURATION:** 35 mins—2 rounds, 55 min—3 rounds

**NOTES:** Perform exercises as a circuit following the prescribed work and rest times.

| EXERCISE | WORK | REST |
|---|---|---|
| 1. Speed Step-Ups | 10 sec | 10 sec |
| 2. Burpees | 20 sec | 20 sec |
| 3. Pushup with Alternating Reach | 30 sec | 30 sec |
| 4. Sumo Squat | 40 sec | 40 sec |
| 5. Toe Touches | 50 sec | 50 sec |
| 6. Alternating Reverse Lunges | 60 sec | 60 sec |

*Rest 30 seconds and repeat x 2-3 rounds*

| REST 2 MINUTES BETWEEN CIRCUITS | | |
|---|---|---|
| 1. Squat Drops | 60 sec | 60 sec |
| 2. Jump Rope | 50 sec | 50 sec |
| 3. Stability Ball Mountain Climbers | 40 sec | 40 sec |
| 4. Stability Ball Leg Curls | 30 sec | 30 sec |
| 5. Scissor Jumps | 20 sec | 20 sec |
| 6. Close Grip Pushups | 10 sec | 10 sec |

*Rest 20 seconds and repeat x 2-3 rounds*

# SPEED STEP-UPS

1. Find a step about 6 inches in height.

2. Alternate stepping up and down on the step as fast as you can. Try to stay light, quick, and on the balls of your feet.

3. Switch your lead foot halfway through your set and repeat.

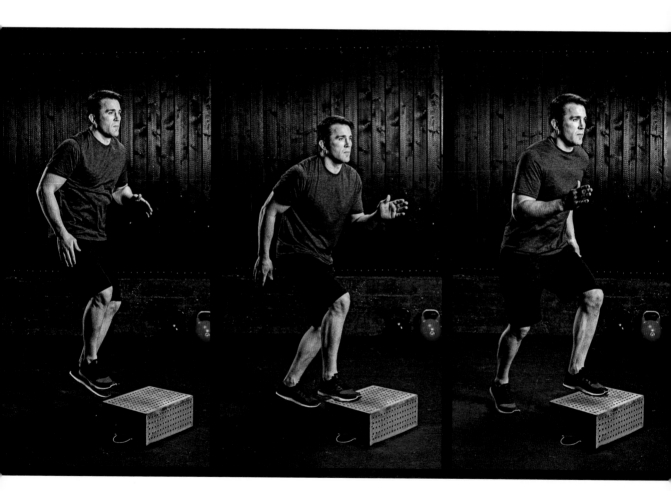

# BURPEES

1. Stand with your feet hip width apart and your arms by your sides.

2. Lower into a squat position with your hands flat on the floor in front of you.

3. Kick your legs back so when your feet land you are in a plank position.

4. Lower your chest to the floor with good pushup form.

5. Push back up to the plank position and jump both feet forward so you are back in the squat position.

6. Jump up and raise both hands over your head.

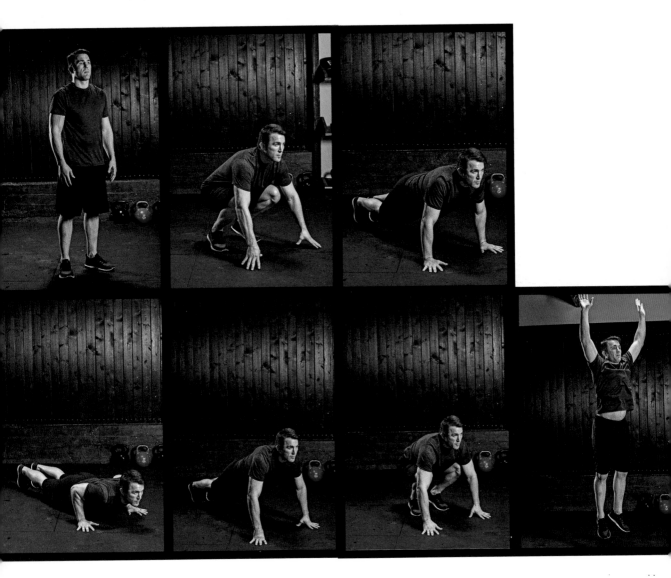

# PUSHUP WITH ALTERNATING REACH

1. Start in plank position, making sure your hips are in line with your ankles and your body forms a straight line.

2. Lower yourself to the bottom of a pushup.

3. As you press back to the top of your pushup, reach your left hand out in front so it's parallel to the floor.

4. Return the left hand to its original plank position, perform another pushup, and reach out with the right hand.

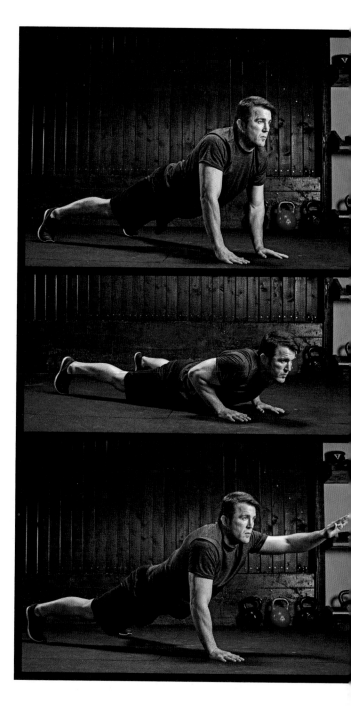

## SUMO SQUAT

1. Stand with your feet in a wide stance, wider than hip-width apart, and angle your toes out.

2. Bend your knees and hips to lower into your squat, squeezing your glutes at the bottom of the move. Arms rise to horizontal for stability.

3. Do not allow your knees to go out beyond your toes or your torso to lean forward. Keep your back neutral and long, drawing the tailbone straight down to the floor each time.

4. Once lowered, drive through your heels back to standing.

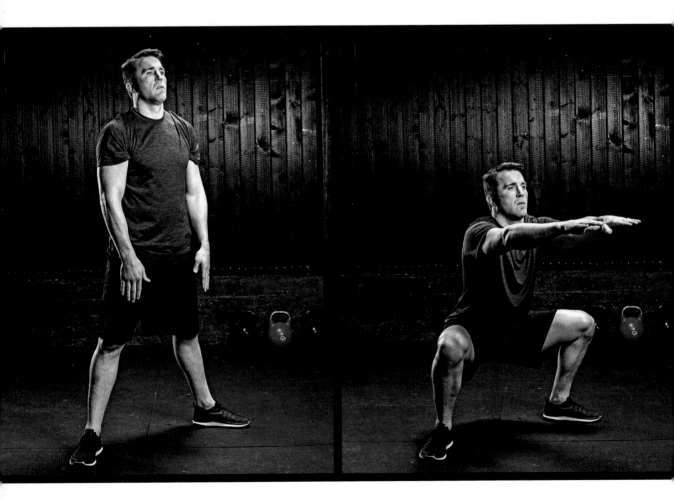

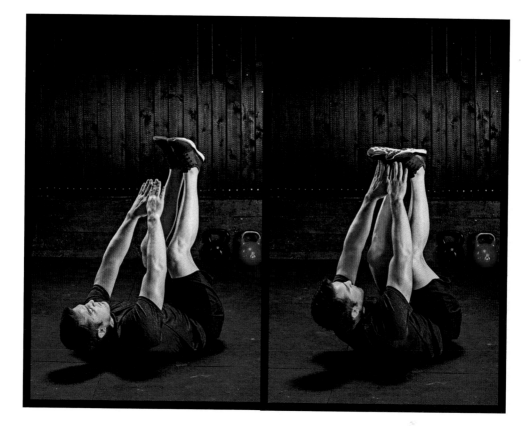

## TOE TOUCHES

1. To begin, lie down with your back pressed against the floor and your legs touching each other. Your arms should reach out from your sides with the palms facing down.

2. Slowly elevate your legs in the air until they are almost perpendicular to the floor with a slight bend at the knees. Your feet should be parallel to the floor.

3. Reach your arms up so they are fully extended and also perpendicular to the floor. This is the starting position.

4. While keeping your lower back pressed against the floor, slowly lift your chest and use your hands to try and touch your toes. Remember to exhale while perform this part of the exercise. Do not reach with your neck.

5. Slowly lower your torso and arms back down to the starting position while inhaling. Remember to keep your arms straight, pointing toward your toes.

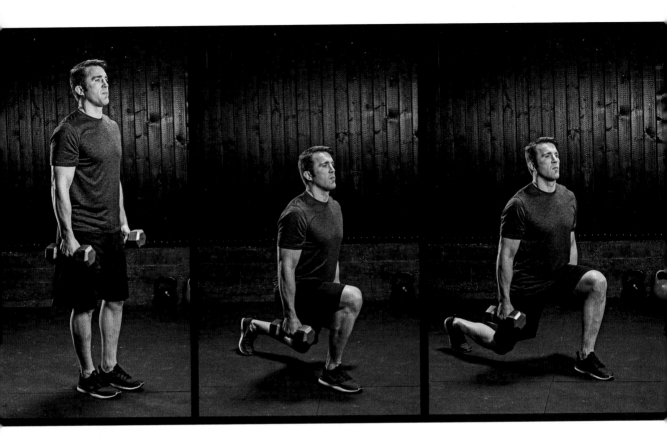

## ALTERNATING REVERSE LUNGES

1. Stand tall with your feet together and hands at your hips or hanging at your sides with weights in your hands.

2. Take a large and controlled step back with your left foot.

3. Lower your left knee (back leg) to the ground, lightly touching the floor, while maintaining your torso upright and your weight slightly more on the front leg.

4. Keep your right knee just above your ankle.

5. Return to standing by pressing your right heel into the floor and bringing your left leg forward to complete one rep.

6. Alternate legs and step back with the right.

# SQUAT DROPS

1. Start in a standing position with your feet shoulder width apart and your hands by your sides.

2. Drop down quickly into a deep squat position. Hands may be clasped or by your side.

3. As you stand back up tall, hop in the air, bringing your legs together and touching your feet together, then immediately drop back into the squat positon and repeat the movement.

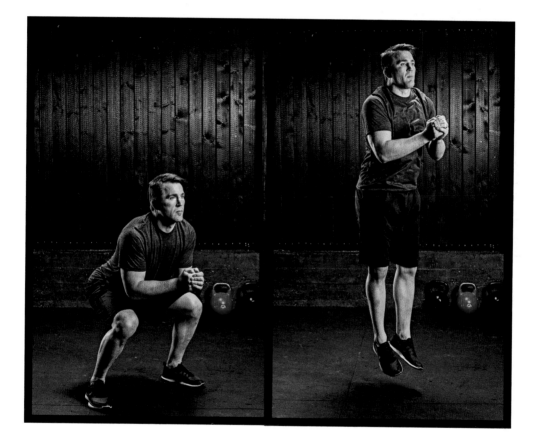

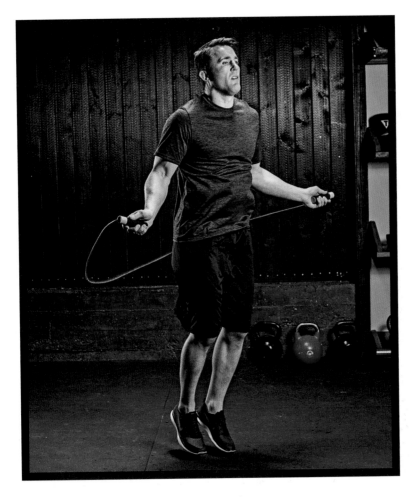

## JUMP ROPE

1. Stand with your feet about hip width apart, gripping a handle of the jump rope in each hand. Your thumbs should be pointed away from your sides.

2. Swing the rope over your head from back to front. As the rope comes around, jump over it.

3. Keep the momentum of the rope going as you jump each time.

# STABILITY BALL MOUNTAIN CLIMBERS

1. Begin in a pushup plank position with your hands on the ball at shoulder width apart.

2. Tighten your abdominal muscles and slowly raise your right knee toward your chest.

3. Control the stability ball by keeping tension in your chest and core.

4. Return your right leg back to the starting position.

5. Alternate legs quickly but while remaining in control.

6. This is identical to the mountain climbers described previously, except you're now stabilizing the ball with your hands instead of your hands on the ground.

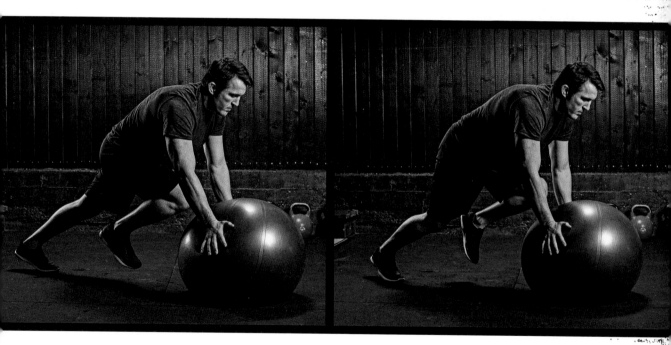

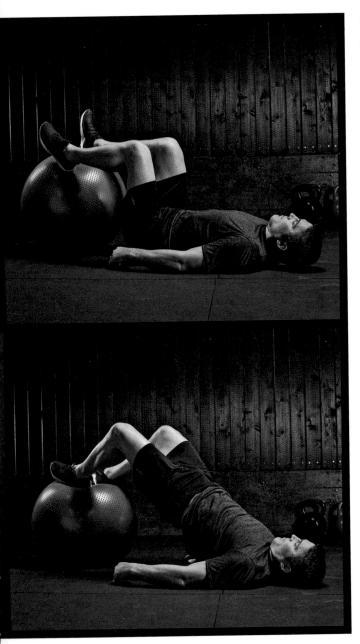

## STABILITY BALL LEG CURLS

1. Begin on the floor, lying on your back with your legs extended and your ankles resting on top of the ball. Your arms should be at your sides, palms down.

2. Raise your hips off the ground, keeping your weight on your shoulder blades and your feet.

3. Bend your knees, pulling the ball as close to you as you can by contracting your hamstrings.

4. After a brief pause, return to the starting position.

# SCISSOR JUMPS

1. Start in a lunge position with your right foot forward and your left leg back with your knee a few inches from the floor.

2. Explosively jump up and switch leg positions while in the air, so both feet land at the same time but now with your left foot in front and your right foot behind.

3. Bend your knees as you land and allow your leg muscles to absorb and control the landing. Then explosively jump up again and repeat.

4. Continue jumping and alternating legs.

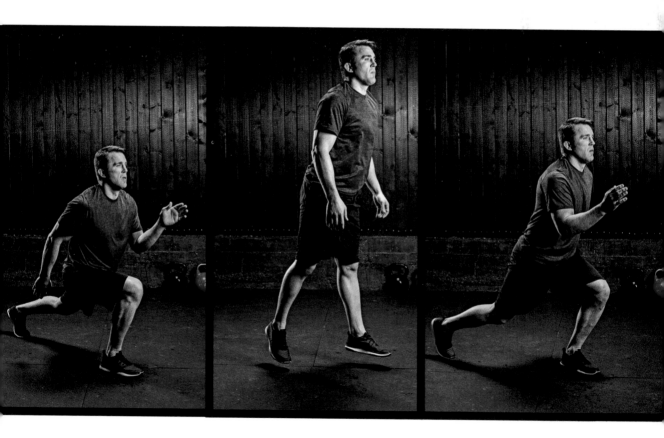

# CLOSE-GRIP PUSHUPS

1. Get into a pushup plank position, but place your hands closer than shoulder width (6 to 10 inches apart) into a "close-grip" position. Make sure you keep good pushup form, keeping core tension and holding your body in a straight line.

2. Lower yourself as you inhale, keeping your elbows tight to your body along your ribs until your chest touches or almost touches the floor.

3. Press your upper body back to the starting position and squeeze your chest. Breathe out as you perform this step.

4. After a pause at the top, repeat the movement for the prescribed amount of repetitions.

5. If you can't perform on the floor, elevate your hands on a box, bench, or stationary bar to put less weight on your arms. Follow the same guidelines.

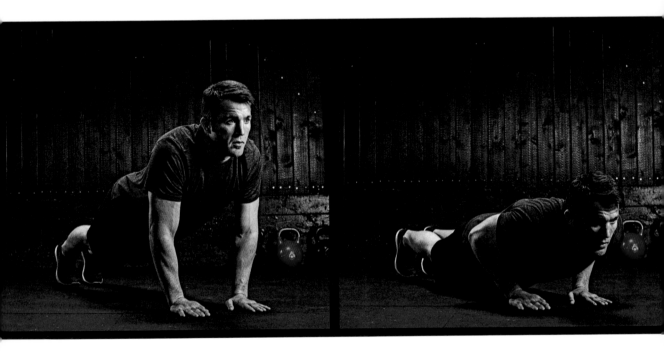

## WORKOUT 4: AMRAP (As Many Rounds As Possible)

**EQUIPMENT NEEDED:** 12–18-inch box, 2 dumbbells, 1 kettlebell

**ESTIMATED DURATION:** 15–25 minutes

**NOTES:** Perform exercises as a continuous circuit, completing as many rounds as possible.

| EXERCISE | REPS |
|---|---|
| 1. Box Jumps (or Squat Jumps) | 5 |
| 2. Single-Arm Dumbbell Row | 10 each |
| 3. Kettlebell Swings | 10 |
| 4. Pushups | 10 |
| 5. Alternating V-Ups | 20 |
| 6. Lunge Walks | 20 |
| 7. Lateral Line Hops | 30 |
| 8. Jump Rope | 50 |

*Back to the top and repeat AMRAP (As Many Rounds As Possible)*

# BOX JUMPS (OR SQUAT JUMPS)

1. Stand with your feet shoulder width apart, about a foot behind a small (12–18-inch) box.

2. Drop quickly into a quarter squat, then extend your hips, swing your arms, and push your feet through the floor to propel yourself onto the box.

3. Land soft in a slight squat position.

4. Choose a box that you can easily jump onto. The goal is not to pull your knees and feet up onto a high box, but to jump OVER the box and land controlled on top of it.

5. Always step back down controlled to the start position. NEVER jump back off the box.

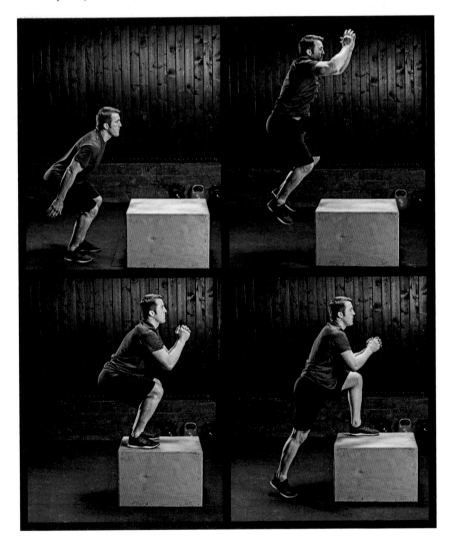

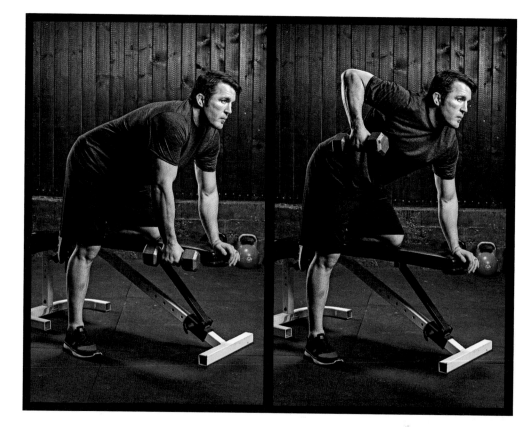

## SINGLE-ARM DUMBBELL ROW

1. Choose a flat bench and place a dumbbell on each side of it.

2. Place your left knee on the bench at one end. Hinge your chest forward from the waist until your upper body is parallel to the floor. Place your left hand on the other end of the bench for support and drive into the floor with your right foot.

3. Use the right hand to pick up the dumbbell on the floor and hold the weight while keeping your lower back straight. The palm of your right hand should face the bench.

4. Pull the dumbbell straight up to the side of your chest, keeping your upper arm close to your side.

5. Lower the dumbbell straight down to the starting position. Breathe in as you perform this step.

6. Repeat on the opposite side by switching which knee is on the bench and using the other dumbbell, which you have already placed into position.

## KETTLEBELL SWINGS

See page 98.

## PUSH-UPS

See page 95.

## ALTERNATING V-UPS

1. Lie on your back with your legs straight and your arms extended on the floor above your head.

2. Bring your opposite arm and leg up to touch in the air above you.

3. Return to your starting position.

4. Repeat with your other arm and leg. Each time your hand has touched both your left and right leg equals one repetition.

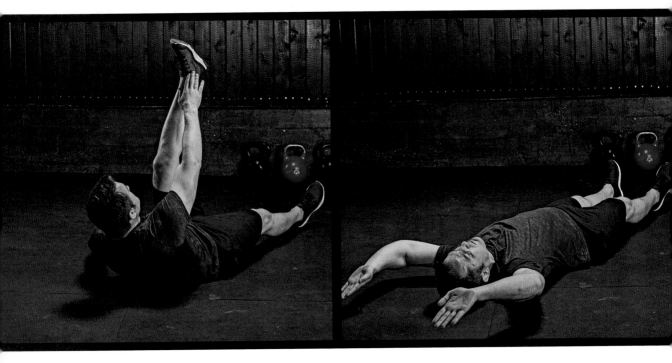

# LUNGE WALKS

1.  Begin standing with your feet shoulder width apart and your hands on your hips.

2.  Step forward with your left leg, bending your knees to drop your hips. Descend until your rear knee (your right knee) nearly touches the ground. Once here, your posture should remain upright and your front knee should be aligned above the front foot.

3.  Drive through the heel of your left foot and extend both knees to raise yourself back up.

4.  Step forward with your rear/right foot, repeating the lunge on the right leg.

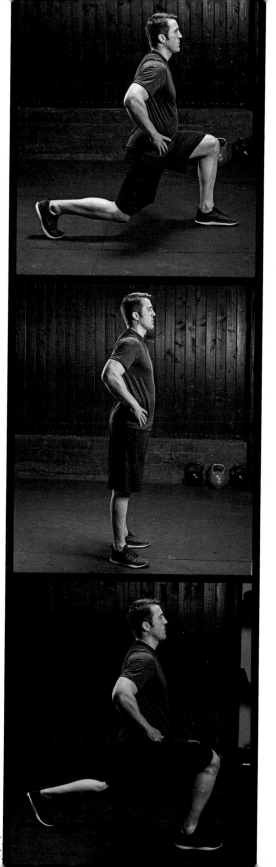

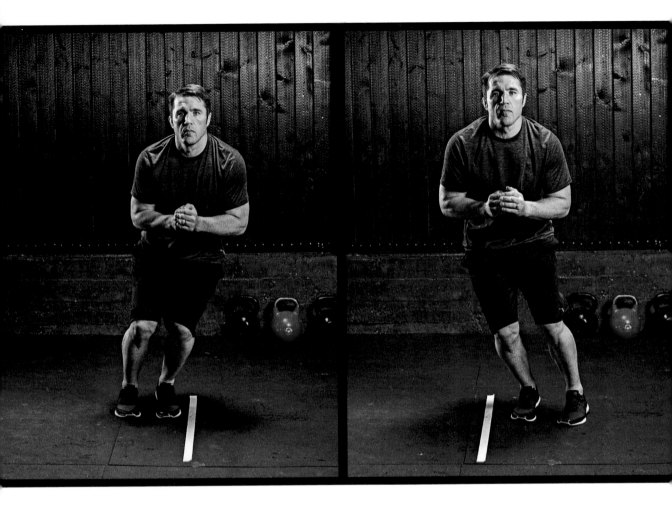

## LATERAL LINE HOPS

1. Start in an athletic position (butt back, knees bent, chest forward) on one side of a tape line.
2. Perform quick hops on the balls of your feet, jumping side to side over the line.
3. Stand up tall, keeping your knees bent and in line with your feet.
4. Perform this exercise as quickly as you are able without losing proper technique.

## JUMP ROPE

See page 126.

## How to Improve Your Flexibility

Being flexible lies at the heart of the Four-Pack Revolution. Moving fluidly with ease makes sitting in front of the computer or fighting in a cage easier. With aging, the discs in your spine lose fluid and begin to shrink. Joint range of motion decreases, muscles become less elastic, and your metabolism slows. How sad. But you can do something about it! Ryan's mother first achieved her legs splits at age 50! You have no excuses.

The masters of strength and flexibility are gymnasts. They achieve an unbelievable balance between these two physical attributes by making both a priority. The stretching they do isn't overly complicated, though. They just stretch frequently and are willing to endure some discomfort while holding uncomfortable positions. Just like losing weight, consistency and a little sacrifice also apply to flexibility. Your body will respond.

The basics of safe, effective stretching apply to everyone, whether you're young, old, fat, or thin.

- **Stretch when your body is warm:** You'll get better results when your blood is flowing. You can warm up with a walk around the block, some jumping jacks, or more complex exercises. Just do something to get your blood flowing before stretching.

- **Stay pain-free:** Stretching is not the time to show how tough you are. Tension is good as long as you breathe through it, but pain is not. Your body knows the difference.

- **Form counts:** Stretching is a great time to listen to your body. Where are the restrictions? What is not quite right? Keeping good form helps prevent injury and allows you to both master the positions and measure progress.

- **Start slow and hold the position:** No bouncing necessary. Focus on your breath as you imagine yourself opening up. The longer you hold each position, the better.

- **Stretch regularly:** Consistency is key. Every time you make the effort to stretch is a check in the win column.

Ideally, stretching should be part of your daily routine. The floor in front of your television is one of the best places to improve your flexibility. Stretching your hamstrings and back for just 5 minutes can help alleviate restrictions that contribute to chronic pain. A jump band (think: giant rubber band) also makes stretching easy and fun. The longer you hold the positions, the better the results will be.

While you're stretching, it is important to focus on your breathing. You may want to practice proper breathing separately in order to master the basics. Here's how to practice "yoga breathing," which is what we suggest you do during your stretching sessions.

1. Sit or lie down in a comfortable position, with your hands gently resting on your lower abs.

2. Focus your attention on your breathing. Inhale through your nose and feel your hands rise with your abdomen with each breath.

3. Hold each breath for a count of five, then slowly exhale through your mouth as your abs return to their resting position.

4. As you improve, work to increase the exhalation time with the aim of making this phase of your breathing twice as long as inhalation.

5. Once you have become comfortable with your breathing, incorporate these deep breaths into your stretching routine. You will be surprised how much they impact your flexibility while calming the mind.

## System Reset

Your hormones and metabolism will function at their peak on workout days. The harder you go, the more efficient your body will become. You can take advantage of this on your System Reset day. A challenging training session will help your body process the overload of calories, sugar, and fat. So if you plan to have a System Reset meal, schedule your hardest workout for the same day.

## OVERVIEW

Many people mistakenly assume that spending an hour on the treadmill will shed those pounds. Yes, you will burn calories, but you can't exercise enough to compensate for a poor diet. Ironically, if you did manage to work out long enough, your appetite would sky-rocket and you'd end up in a food–exercise arms race. The pace would be impossible to sustain, your risk of injury would increase, and if you slowed down, chances are you would keep eating the same amount and gaining weight as a result. Remember, the purpose of exercise is to build muscle, reduce stress, improve sleep, and regulate hormones.

## QUICK-START GUIDE

Everyone starts somewhere. This time, let's get started in a way that sets you up for long-term success. The goal is to start creating new habits while utilizing positive results as a source of motivation. The three areas to leverage are food, exercise, and the way you're thinking about your problems. As you begin, find one or two small adjustments to make as you begin to turn things around.

### Diet Jumpstarts

Losing weight can seem daunting, especially if it's been a source of chronic pain and frustration for you. But don't despair.

- **Go-to meals:** Do you know why people watch their favorite movies over and over again? It's a guaranteed good time. You can re-create a similar experience with food. Having four or five enjoyable, go-to meals in your arsenal makes sticking to the plan that much easier. With fewer variables to account for, you can monitor your progress while making small adjustments along the way.

- **Calorie shaving:** Shaving calories is all about making minor adjustments to reduce calories that don't affect the taste of a meal. For example, try using a teaspoon of oil instead of a tablespoon. This saves 80 calories that you probably won't miss. Eating a small handful of nuts versus diving into the jar of nut butter with a spoon will save even more. Over time, these small efforts add up.

### Workouts

If you're new to working out or it's been a while, don't rush in. The exercises in each workout are not difficult, but give yourself time to learn the technique. In the long term this will reduce your chance of injury. Your body loves variety, and sometimes you may not feel like training hard. When you're not in the mood for an intense workout, it makes sense to have a lighter day.

- If you're overweight and out of shape, it's best to start slow—remember, small victories. Get used to moving your body again and appreciate the freedom that movement brings.

- If you're recovering from injury or illness, you may not want to push yourself too hard until you are fully recovered. Save your energy for the healing process.

- If you are tired from a long week and don't have the motivation to work out, then a long walk is the perfect activity to burn a few calories and decrease stress.

## FOUR-WEEK QUICK START

We're going to get you started over with our Four-Week Quick Start training plan. These workouts can be as easy or difficult as you make them and do not require much time or equipment. Each Four-Pack strength and conditioning workout was created by master trainer P.J. Nestler and is designed to improve range of motion, decrease body fat, and build lean muscle while strengthening your heart and lungs.

### Self-Check

Obstacles and distractions are a part of life. There will be occasions when you drift off course, finding yourself repeating old patterns or just feeling like things will never change. Expect this, as it's part of the process. What isn't okay is thinking you shouldn't have any problems. Problems are not the problem; your response to life's challenges and successes is what matters most. When you find yourself wondering what to do next, any one of these tips will serve as a compass to lead you back in the right direction. None of them take long or require much planning or effort.

Keeping yourself in check is a big responsibility. It can be a dirty job, but someone has to do it. Since only you are responsible for you, you'll need to take the lead. When you run into a challenge, start by asking yourself these three questions.

1. Am I part of the solution or part of the problem?

2. How do I want to look back at today 10 years from now?

3. What are three small changes I can make right now to regain control and move myself in the direction of my dreams?

## STOP COMPLAINING

Victims complain, and whining robs us of our ability to effectively navigate a challenge. Why? People complain when they are in pain, when they feel powerless in a situation and don't know what to do about it. Sometimes it's just a bad habit we fall into. Start paying close attention to your thoughts and the words that come out of your mouth, as they impact the quality of your life. The next time you catch yourself in victim mode, drop and do 10 pushups. This will increase your awareness and help break the pattern.

## ARE YOUR STANDARDS TOO HIGH?

Frustration appears when life isn't going to plan. Unrealistic expectations increase the intensity of these emotions, which leads to poor decisions. We all need to reevaluate the standards to which we hold ourselves and those around us to from time to time. When the bar is set so high you can never reach it, all you've done is guarantee failure.

## AVOID ALL OR NONE

Some days won't be your best, so avoid the negative trap of "all or nothing" thinking. Bad days happen to everyone; give yourself permission to join the rest of us. Sometimes a victory is simply not going completely off the rails. Any amount you can reel things back in is a step forward. Remember: Strive for excellence, not perfection.

## SCHEDULE FAILURE

If you're the type of person who loves to go all in and it has been months since you've deviated from your perfect diet, pick your favorite restaurant or meal and go for it. Often, those who take an absolute approach will achieve incredible results in the short term, but their pace and intensity are impossible to sustain. When the pendulum starts to swing, they go just as hard in the opposite direction.

## System Reset Meal Management

As we mentioned earlier, you're going to be eating several times a day, every day, for the rest of your life. On occasion, some of those meals aren't going to be entirely healthy. No problem. Done properly, a System Reset meal can curb cravings with few negative consequences. However, eating unhealthy food can be a slippery slope, so make sure you keep it in perspective. Here are a few suggestions to minimize any negative effect from a System Reset meal.

- **Work out:** System Reset meals should coincide with your most intense workout of the week. This will put your body in the best position to process the food. Strength training on these days helps considerably, and if you really want to tame that meal, add a second workout a few hours after eating.

- **Keep each meal in perspective:** The most important tip for minimizing any negative effects of your System Reset meal is to not have two in a row. Be one and done until the following week. These meals are an exception to the rule, and the healthier and leaner you are, the more efficiently you'll process these foods.

## Small Victories

The backbone of long-term success is small victories. The seemingly insignificant decisions you make on a daily basis are the biggest predictor of how far you will go. During busy or stressful times, it can be easy to lose sight of the power of this approach. Below is a list of ideas that will help you maintain momentum.

- **Keep the motor running:** Do 50 squats after each meal. A little activity after meals will improve the digestive process and improve how well your cells absorb nutrients from the bloodstream.

- **Take a walk:** If you're too busy to get a workout in, go for a walk. This is a trick we use when cutting weight for a fight. A walk at the end of the day doesn't take much energy, it's low stress, it burns calories, and it refreshes the mind. Plus it keeps you from snacking.

- **Do the dishes:** Completing a task that improves your life is empowering. It reminds you that you have control of your actions and can use them to improve your life at any time. This is the same principle I used while running up the stairs in my house when I was beginning to get back in shape. Doing something positive and completing the task sends a message to your brain that you are ready for change.

- **Breathe:** Stress is a major contributor to an unhealthy lifestyle, and when we're under stress most of us forget to breathe properly. The best role models we have for healthy breathing are babies and puppies. They are like yoga masters, utilizing their diaphragm with each deep breath. Download relaxation or guided imagery soundtracks on your phone, and use them whenever your blood pressure starts to rise.

- **Floss your teeth:** Dental problems can contribute to low-grade inflammation in your body. All the more reason to floss. Most people don't like eating with a fresh, clean mouth, so a well-timed brushing can help you forget about food cravings in the moment. Even if this doesn't work, you've still improved your dental hygiene. One more small victory.

- **Use a smaller plate:** It may sound a little strange, but chances are you'll eat less if your plate is smaller. There's even scientific research that backs this up. If you're fresh out of small plates, get into the habit of leaving some food on your plate. It may seem wasteful at first, but this really is a better option than shoving excess calories down your throat. You can always feed your leftovers to the dog.

## FOUR-WEEK WORKOUT CALENDAR

| | DAY 1 | DAY 2 | DAY 3 | |
|---|---|---|---|---|
| **Week 1** | **CORE CARDIO** Time: 20 min | **STRENGTH & METABOLIC** Time: 30-45 min | **STEADY STATE CARDIO*** Time: 45-60 min | |
| **Week 2** | **STRENGTH & METABOLIC** Time: 20 min | **STEADY STATE CARDIO*** Time: 30-45 min | **PYRAMID** Time: 45-60 min | |
| **Week 3** | **CORE CARDIO** Time: 20 min | **AMARP** Time: 30-45 min | **STEADY STATE CARDIO*** Time: 45-60 min | |
| **Week 4** | **PYRAMID** Time: 20 min | **STEADY STATE CARDIO*** Time: 30-45 min | **STRENGTH & METABOLIC** Time: 45-60 min | |

- **Revisit your diet plan:** If you keep running into the same problems, examine your diet and make a few small changes. Maybe you need a little less carbs and more vegetables, or perhaps those System Reset meals are starting to happen daily. Whatever it is, if you pay closer attention to what you're eating, you'll quickly find areas to improve.

- **Snack before going out to dinner:** That basket of warm bread taunting you as your server takes too long to come back to the table can be tough to ignore. A small snack before you arrive at the restaurant can help take the edge off. A handful of nuts, a low-sugar Greek yogurt, or a low-calorie protein shake are all great options.

- **Clear out the kitchen:** If there's temptation in the house, get rid of it. Don't make it easy for yourself to fail. It's impossible to eat a pint of chocolate ice cream if it's not in your freezer. Are you going to drive to the store at 10 p.m. to pick some up? Probably not, especially if you have other, healthier options in your kitchen.

| DAY 4 | DAY 5 | DAY 6 | DAY 7 |
|---|---|---|---|
| **PYRAMID** | **CORE CARDIO** | **AMARP** | |
| Time: 30-45 min | Time: 20 min | Time: 30-45 | Active Rest |
| **CORE CARDIO** | **STRENGTH & METABOLIC** | **STEADY STATE CARDIO*** | |
| Time: 30-45 min | Time: 20 min | Time: 30-45 | Active Rest |
| **PYRAMID** | **CORE CARDIO** | **STRENGTH & METABOLIC** | |
| Time: 30-45 min | Time: 20 min | Time: 30-45 | Active Rest |
| **CORE CARDIO** | **AMARP** | **STEADY STATE CARDIO*** | |
| Time: 30-45 min | Time: 20 min | Time: 30-45 | Active Rest |

- **Pack a snack:** Don't get caught in a situation where you're hungry and have nothing but unhealthy food to eat. Pack a few healthy snacks that you can turn to when those cravings kick in. The masters of snack packing are moms. They know how a few calories can stave off negative emotions, i.e., getting "hangry." The same approach that works for kids will work for you.

- **Take a nap:** If you're tired, everything in life becomes more difficult. Sleep is the cornerstone of controlling your weight. It impacts the hormones that control how you burn and store fat, and the better your hormones work, the more effective your weight management will be. An afternoon nap is popular in many places in the world, and there are companies in the United States putting nap rooms into their corporate headquarters. A 20-minute power nap can provide the boost you need to finish your day strong.

- **Get up:** Do you spend most of your day sitting at a desk? In 2015, a report published in the *Annals of Internal Medicine* found the average American spends more

*Steady state cardio involves exercising with a continuous, steady effort. Use the talk test during your workout—if you can carry on a conversation while exercising you're in the right place.

than half the day sitting. At a desk, in a car, or on the couch, sitting contributes to heart disease, decreased metabolism, and back and hip pain. As a human being, you come from a long line of hunter-gatherers. Your body was designed to move efficiently in your environment, not to sit still. A standing desk has been shown to increase productivity by 46 percent. With many inexpensive options available—including simply piling a bunch of books on your existing desk—it's something worth looking into.

# 7
# WINNING
# MINDSET

## OAKLAND, CALIFORNIA, AUGUST 7, 2010

There I was—one round to go, just five minutes away from realizing a lifelong goal of becoming a world champion. I had just spent 20 minutes on top of UFC champion Anderson Silva, ground-and-pounding my way to victory. I was a little bit surprised by how easily I'd been able to dominate him. Round after round I took him down, put him on his back, and proceeded to punch him until the bell rang. With five short minutes left on the clock, things were looking good for Uncle Chael.

If you don't know the backstory, here's the short version. Anderson Silva was the most dominant champion in UFC history and had reached almost mythical status in his native Brazil. Now, I didn't have anything against him personally, but he had something I wanted. So I spent the better part of a year tormenting him in the media every chance I had. Each time I won a fight in the UFC, I only mentioned Silva's name during the post-fight interview. It was only a matter of time until I got my shot.

By the time the bell rang, UFC 117 had become the largest gate in UFC history and our fight was broadcast in 173 territories and countries. Despite receiving numerous death threats from Brazil, I was exactly where I wanted to be. As the underdog, not many pundits were predicting I would win. But from the moment the fight began, it was clear that I had the upper hand. This was a five-round fight, and for four rounds I beat him up and dominated in every way possible and the crowd was loving it. They were so loud I had trouble hearing my cornermen speak between rounds. The fifth and final round went exactly as the previous four did—until the very end, when I lost focus for a brief moment and Silva executed a perfect triangle choke. Game over. This lack of focus cost me a world championship and millions of dollars. Sometimes life doesn't go as planned.

## FAILURE IS ALWAYS AN OPTION

Dealing with setbacks, real or imagined, is an underdeveloped skill for many of us. As a result, two scenarios occur. Either the fear of failure becomes so strong it prevents us from even starting, or we implode from losses because the pain is too great to bear. But failure is always an option—for everyone. Those inspirational posters featuring a rock climber hanging from a cliff by one hand with the slogan "failure is not an option" are false. You *can* fail. You have failed in the past and you will fail again in the future. So you had better learn to come out the other side stronger, or you'll never come close to realizing your true potential. Because there's a flip side to failure that's often overlooked: Our blunders create valuable opportunities for learning that we miss when celebrating our successes.

By now you must realize that you can't be in peak shape all year round. But this isn't the real problem. The struggle of managing the off times, where your weight increases and your motivation lags, is where the battle is won or lost. Holidays represent the most obvious pitfall. Summer is over, the weather is getting cooler, and there are numerous opportunities to overeat. How can you respond to the natural cycles we all go through so that your weight doesn't spin out of control? In the 2011 American Psychological Association's annual Stress in America™ survey, 27 percent of respondents blamed lack of willpower as their most significant barrier to change. "If only I had more willpower. . . ." As if willpower is some mystical force that will magically solve your problems.

## Willpower vs. Strategy

Willpower gets a bad rap, mostly because we expect it to help in ways it was never equipped to do. Think of it this way: Willpower is akin to the afterburner on a fighter jet, used to get the aircraft rapidly up to speed before relying on the main engines to achieve continuous momentum. Afterburners are powerful in the moment, but require a lot of fuel. If they are relied on for too long, the plane will rapidly run out of gas. Like afterburners, willpower is a valuable resource as long as it's used properly—in short bursts, as a powerful fuel source to stay on track. It's not designed to carry you through to the promised land.

Strategy is what fuels long-term success. It accounts for contingencies, anticipates potential pitfalls, and helps navigate the myriad unexpected problems that inevitably pop up. Anticipating what can go wrong isn't being negative—it's being smart. Successful coaches do this routinely when creating a game plan for an upcoming match. Acknowledging an opponent's strengths and their athlete's weaknesses helps prepare for the unexpected. Similarly, understanding portion size, how macronutrients contribute to weight loss, and identifying the best ways to include exercise in your daily schedule are all components of building an effective and achievable strategy for achieving a four-pack.

## What Does an Ancient Chinese Military General Know about Losing Weight?

Sun Tzu–the ancient Chinese general, military strategist, and philosopher–wrote the book *The Art of War* 2,500 years ago. This influential military strategy book is still used today by athletes and executives looking to gain an advantage. The lessons in Sun Tzu's book are simple, and apply to your health and weight-loss goals as well.

1.  **Opportunities multiply as they are seized.** Sun Tzu understood the power of momentum and how one success leads to another. Each opportunity you seize reinforces new habits. Even the shortest workout or the smallest change in your diet has value. Take time to consider your options and look for small wins to build momentum.

2.  **Avoid what is strong. Attack what is weak.** Find easy wins. It's the quickest way to build momentum and self-confidence. You can always tackle tougher challenges in the future. If a healthy snack reduces cravings and makes driving past the drive-thru window at a fast food restaurant easier, then do it. You'll have moved yourself forward.

3.  **Victorious warriors win first and then go to war, while defeated warriors go to war first and then seek to win.** Preparation determines success. Expecting you'll reach your goals by figuring out everything in the moment is a recipe for failure. This is one more reason not to rush this weight-loss process. Stop, and consider what didn't work in the past and what your options are moving forward.

4.  **If the mind is willing, the flesh could go on and on without many things.** Sun Tzu was a master at motivating his troops and knew that if they were engaged with a purpose, their chances of success were much greater. Inspiring goals generate energy and make resisting temptation easier. Remember, your mind is much stronger than you may give it credit for.

5.  **According as circumstances are favorable, one should modify one's plans.** The need to be flexible and respond to a changing environment was as important on the battlefield 2,500 years ago as it is today. Don't let your standards slip because something unexpected happens. Remain flexible and adapt.

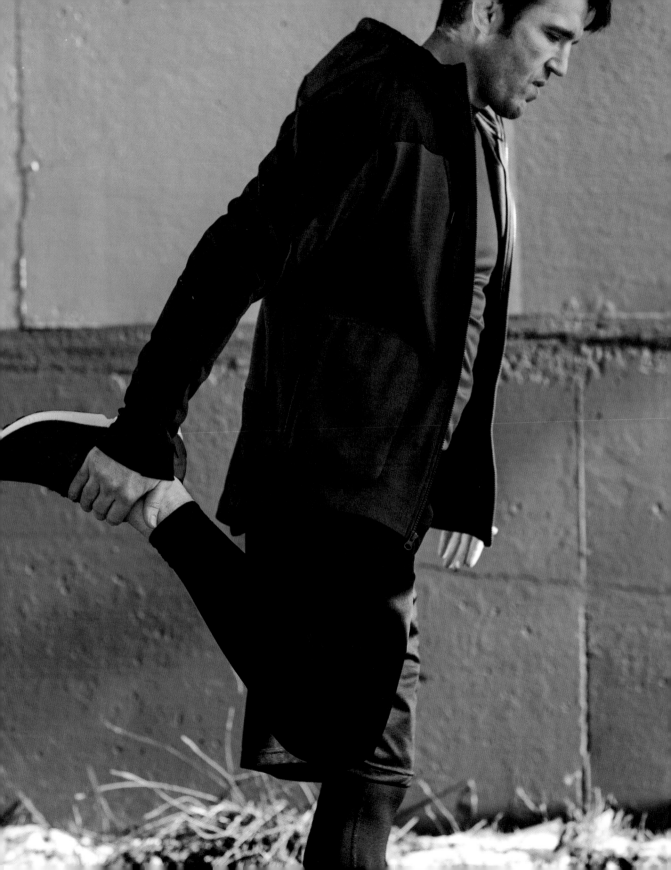

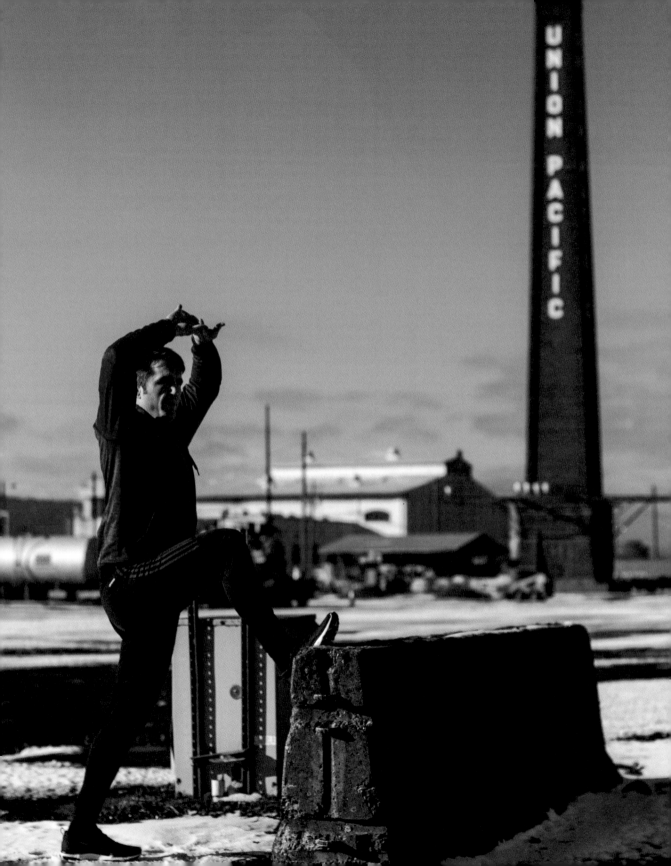

## Expect to Win

"It's not that you won or lost, but how you played the game." Um, what? Yes, winning does matter. It's important. Once you experience it, you'll want more. But if you've suffered failures in the past, it can be easy to let that inner voice of doubt grow louder. Even elite athletes are not immune to this, and climbing out of a slump can present a real challenge. Just ask Tiger Woods. But without at least a suspicion that your goals are possible and a strong belief in your capability to solve any problem, your chances of success decrease significantly.

One of the best examples of a winning mindset comes from UFC fighter Michael Bisping. By his own admission, he's not the strongest, fastest, or most talented athlete in the UFC, but he has a will to win like no one else has. Never one to make excuses, even after losses, he'd return to the gym with an unwavering confidence that he could beat any man on the planet. It turns out Bisping's belief in himself trumped anyone else's view of his capabilities. The man who many fight fans called "pillow fists" knocked out UFC champion Luke Rockhold, took his belt back to England, and eventually tied the record for the most wins in UFC history.

If you're currently in a slump with regard to your weight, go find some easy battles to win to build confidence and increase motivation. That said, you really can louse up your road to victory by aiming too high and expecting immediate results. So keep it simple. A short walk around the block after dinner equals a win. Skipping the drive-thru at McDonald's, another win. Turning the TV off an hour before bedtime, one more check in the win column. How many of these small victories can you rack up in a day?

## The Poison of Perfection: Lower Your Standards

Perfectionists! They wear this title like a badge of honor, when in fact it's the lowest possible standard someone can have for themselves. Why? Perfection is unobtainable, and who wants to play a game you can't win? When one little thing doesn't go according to plan, perfectionists like to take their ball and go home. They often run a pattern of excuses, self-sabotage, and blame, and rarely reach their true potential. It gets worse. In 2014, the *Review of General Psychology* summarized research that linked perfectionism to suicide. Yikes! If you are a perfectionist, listen up—your chance of success is close to zero,

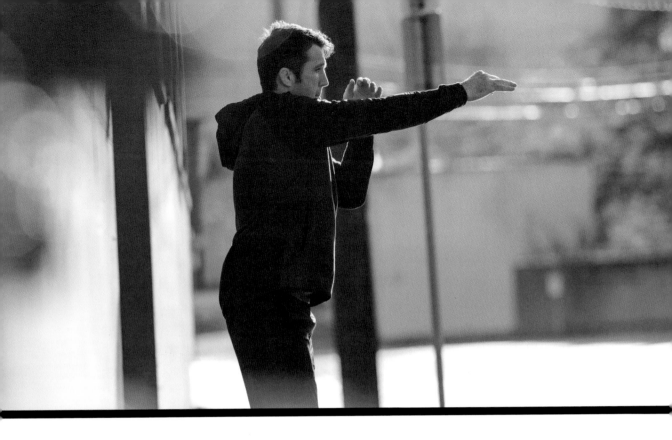

because you will find fault in any achievement. By holding fixed ideas about how life must be, perfectionists miss opportunities and fail to appreciate and learn from their mistakes. They never develop into the people they could be and rarely see the best in others, which strains and occasionally ends relationships. This is no way to live, and is certainly no recipe for achieving your goals.

## WHAT STOPS MOST PEOPLE IS STARTING

When it comes to losing weight, most people fail before they even begin. Unrealistic expectations, unpreparedness, and not having a plan B when plan A stops working all contribute to the high failure rate of dieters. Remember, in order to determine what will work for you, it's essential to know what didn't work in the past. If you're overweight and out of shape, chances are you have made at least one attempt to lose weight. Take a moment to identify what went wrong.

Do you remember what we asked you to do in the introduction? Announce your Four-Pack plans to those around you. Did you do it yet? It's good to put pressure on yourself and have others expect you to live up to your word. Accountability is powerful—we only get better when we're challenged. No one likes to fail; it's disheartening and occasionally embarrassing. Focusing on everything that could (and often will) go wrong is common, but successful people have learned to see past these fears and execute their plans successfully. Fear may still be present, but they have figured out how to compartmentalize their negative emotions and remain calm in the face of uncertainty.

## Start Out Right

Pacing: It's important in marathon races, boxing fights, movie scripts, and weight-loss plans. Yet despite the tremendous level of influence pacing has on our success, it's rarely given much thought. Effective pacing requires forethought and the ability to pass on short-term results in exchange for long-term success. Here are three common strategies that usually implode. Do any of them look familiar?

1. **"Bat Out of Hell"**: A favorite among former athletes—these people pick up right where they left off. Super-focused and intense, they have zero tolerance for failure. In the short term, this approach creates amazing results (or makes someone so sore they don't want to continue). These alphas have no trouble losing 20 pounds in the first month because their focus and hard work are undeniable. But this approach equates to sprinting the first mile of a marathon. Sure, it's easy to be in front of the pack in the beginning, but as time goes by that pace becomes unsustainable. This approach lacks the vision and discipline needed for long-term success.

2. **Doubter**: Doubters may start a new diet or buy a piece of exercise equipment from an infomercial, but there's little conviction behind their actions. They'll play along, for a few weeks anyway. Often, Doubters will join a group of friends who are making the effort they wished they could, but going through the motions without any intensity doesn't produce significant results. Convinced that real change is not possible, why would they bother making the effort?

3. **Planner:** "I'm starting tomorrow" is the mantra. Monday is a Planner's favorite day of the week because it's the start of the latest diet, a cutting-edge workout, and a new life. Weeks, sometimes months are spent researching the perfect meal plan and weight-loss supplements. Special gym equipment is ordered because they can't get in shape without it, but nothing really ever gets going because everything needs to be just right to begin. Planners can easily become perfectionists if they're not careful. While the intent is admirable, this obsession with details is a unique form of procrastination that with each passing Monday grows stronger.

Do any of these well-intentioned strategies look familiar to you? If so, the obvious next question is: How do you break out of that rut? We hear you. You really do want to be successful, but you're just a little confused about how to leave behind those outdated patterns and approach life from a different perspective. Never fear–just keep reading.

## Do It Your Way

After years of elite competition and working with athletes of all levels, it's become quite clear to us there is only one way to be successful–your way. Holly Holm did the impossible when she defeated Ronda Rousey in a classic UFC fight, an achievement very few outside her inner circle thought was possible. Holly is the type of athlete who is always in the gym. She fights on Saturday night and is back to training on Monday morning. This process led her to multiple world titles in boxing and mixed martial arts. Former UFC champion Luke Rockhold takes a different approach: He's known for not doing a lot of training in between fights. A less-is-more approach works better for him. So who is right? The both have big, shiny, UFC championship belts hanging up at home, but their strategies couldn't be more different. Trying to make Luke live Holly's lifestyle would never work, and vice versa. They each adopted an approach to training that matched their individual preferences.

Figuring out what works best for you requires being willing to change your current approach. Remember: pay attention, test, evaluate, and refine. It's a never-ending process.

1.  **Plan for success.** In many ways, successfully navigating a catastrophe is easier than managing the hundreds of minute details required to get through the day. It's often the little things that throw us off track. Planning meals in advance, monitoring your weight, and paying attention to stress put you in a position to achieve positive results.

2.  **Invest.** Any type of success, inward or outward, requires an investment. Exercise is an example that will pay off 4-to-1 in terms of productivity: You'll sleep better, manage stress better, look better, and feel better. But any good investment requires planning, preparation, and sacrifice. Expecting things to just work out is a loser's game. Like a recently retired athlete, you must create new goals to stay motivated.

3.  **Adapt.** Stress, work, or family obligations—this week alone there will be multiple obstacles that get in your way. You must develop the character that allows you to keep progressing toward your goals even when something gets in your way. If you haven't been working out because you loathe commercial gyms, then learn how to swing kettlebells in your garage. If an hour on the treadmill bores you, go play basketball. Convenient options make it easier to adapt. Ryan doesn't like to run. He'll do it, but he's never found it enjoyable. Instead, he put an Air Assault stationary bike in the garage, which provides an effective workout any time of the day. Keeping an open mind and looking for opportunities instead of excuses makes staying on course much easier.

4.  **Have a plan for overcoming procrastination.** Procrastination kills more dreams than methamphetamines. It affects both smart and dumb people, educated and uneducated, the creative and the analytical, and even the rich and poor. When it appears, many people don't even put up a fight. They act like a little submissive dog that flops to his back when an alpha appears. The technical term for procrastination is *akrasia*. It refers to the state of mind in which someone acts against his or her better judgment through weakness of will. Said another way, the root cause of procrastination is an undisciplined mind. The ancient Greek philosopher Aristotle wrote about this 2,300 years ago, so chances are humans have been

procrastinating for as long as there's been something that needed to be done. Strangely enough, most of the tasks we put off doing would take only a few minutes to accomplish. More energy is spent distracting yourself than it would take to sit down, complete the job, and check it off your to-do list.

5. **Pick your battles.** Sun Tzu and Chael are both big believers in this concept. Small victories create momentum, which leads to results. How do you pick your "small battles"? Find one or two easy changes to make that require very little effort. Remember Chael's story about how he got back in shape? He started with one set of stairs in his house. That "workout" could not have taken more than 4 seconds. But it was the beginning that allowed him to build momentum. Six months later, he was down 30 pounds. All too often, people expect to change everything overnight, which only leads to frustration and failure.

6. **Organize your day.** At the start of each fight camp, we write a schedule that serves as a blueprint for everything we hope to accomplish while preparing for the upcoming fight. Fortunately, you don't need this level of detail to lose weight. We've given you workouts, meal plans, recipes, and strategies for putting it all together. Now's the time to start thinking about how you'll use this information. I'm sure there have been times that you've pulled into a drive-thru purely because there were no other readily available options. Consider how you can start avoiding situations where it's easy to eat poorly. Remove temptations from your house and meal prep, because the convenience of processed food can be too tempting to pass up when life gets busy and you get hungry.

7. **Develop discipline.** Discipline is forged by two forces: pain and responsibility. Pain is a great motivator for change, and those uncomfortable emotions carry tremendous energy. When that energy is focused on growth and awareness, a painful experience can lead to extraordinary change. But left on its own, pain fuels unhealthy cycles that lead to frustration and failure. Responsibility transforms victims into leaders who persevere and is the strongest link to self-empowerment. Taking responsibility puts you in the driver's seat while building

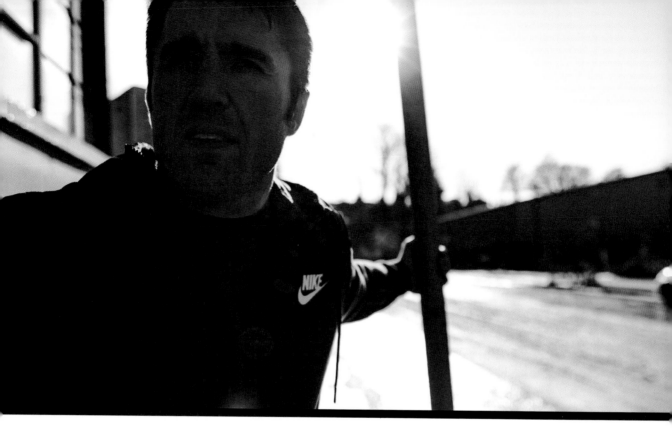

confidence and self-esteem—two essential qualities for anyone looking to take charge of their life.

8.  **Anticipate failure.** Many people have never learned to deal with failure successfully and instead allow their self-worth to be determined by the outcome of an event. When you measure your intrinsic value based on external results, you're in for a rough ride. There's an enlightening book by Steve Young called *Great Failures of the Extremely Successful: Mistakes, Adversity, Failure and Other Steppingstones to Success*. The book is composed of 100 stories of personal failure from highly successful people in all walks of life—business, entertainment, politics, and many more. As unique and varied as each story is, the common thread among them all is massive failure. Each person featured in the book experienced times in their lives when they felt hopeless and didn't know what to do next. But they all went on to live extraordinary lives despite these failures.

There is no way around it–failure is an essential part of the process of becoming successful. Here are a couple of key points to remember when failure happens to you. First, it sucks–you should not like it. But you are not supposed to. Second, remain calm–one slip-up is usually no big deal, especially when it comes to weight loss. It's often the guilt associated with messing up that throws us off track. Third, immediately take a step back in the right direction. Action, aligned with your values and goals, is the only way to turn things around. Lastly, assume responsibility. Yes, some of your problems are your fault. So pack away the blame game, acknowledge your contributions, and get to work.

## SYSTEM RESET

We all need an occasional food break, so let's create a winning mindset in this department as well. When a winner makes a decision, there's no sitting around and feeling guilty about it. If you're going to eat your favorite foods, enjoy them. What's the point if you're going to beat yourself up over one meal? In the first few months, these System Resets are a welcome reprieve. They help keep you from feeling like your dietary challenges will go on forever. Within a short period of time, as you acclimate to your new approach toward healthy living, they won't seem like such a big deal.

## OVERVIEW

Cultivating a winning mindset isn't a weight-loss solution, it's a life solution. Give yourself permission to be the one whose hand is raised at the end. Why not you? At the very least, you should be aware that you're no longer lacking the resources to shed fat, get in shape, and create a four-pack you can be proud of. Physical capability has nothing to do with it. You've made it this far in life, proving your ability to endure tough times, succeeding when the odds were stacked against you. So make the necessary arrangements and expect to win this time around too. In the wise words of Ryan's daughter's gymnastics coach, Coach Brent: "Toughen up, princess."

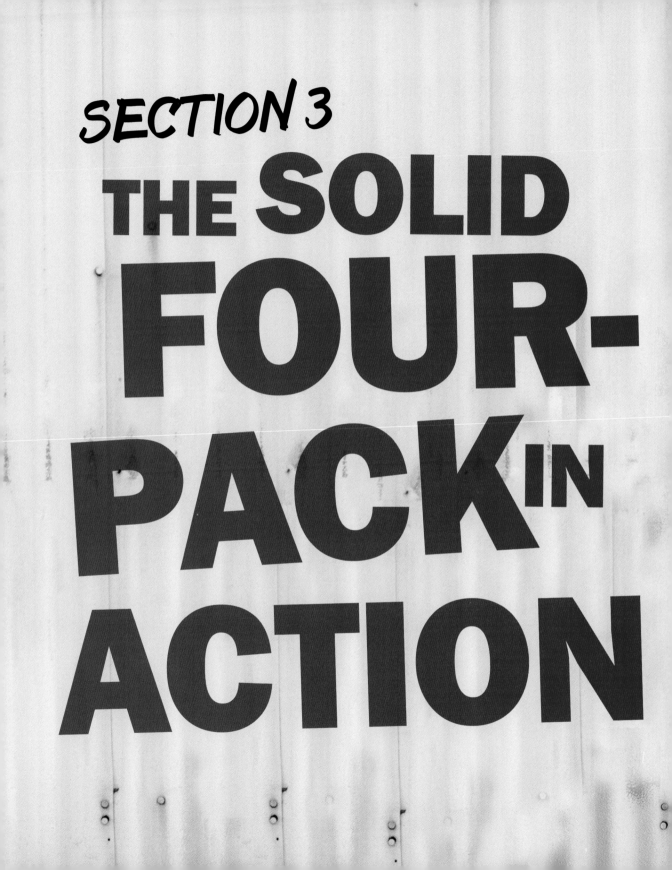

# THE SOLID FOUR-PACK IN ACTION

# 8

# HABITS

**HOW DOES A GOLDFISH
EAT A SHARK? IN A LOT
OF LITTLE BITES**

**I**F YOU'RE AN AMATEUR-WRESTLING FAN, YOU PROBABLY REMEMBER THE NAME Pat Smith, the first four-time NCAA Division I champion. Two of the five losses Pat suffered were to a man named Dan Russell. In addition to being a great athlete himself, Dan understands how to motivate people. Around the time I started to get back in shape, Dan called and shared an inspirational story about his neighbor, who desperately needed to lose weight and was having a heck of a time finding his way. His neighbor was doing what many people do: start, stop, start, stop. Stopping is the one thing guaranteed to kill a deal every time. In business, weight loss, or a fight, you've got to start the clock and keep moving.

So Dan's neighbor wanted to get back in shape and, for whatever reason, couldn't find a way to get it done. Since he was a morning guy, Dan suggested starting his day with an early morning run. But each morning his neighbor found something else to do: sleep in, get dressed, check his email, watch the news—anything but that run. So Dan changed his approach, "Okay, every morning at 6:00 a.m., I want you to put on your workout clothes and walk out to the mailbox. Whatever you do after that is fine; you've succeeded for the day."

Something clicked with this advice, and his neighbor started doing just that. He'd walk outside with his coffee in hand, touch the mailbox, and walk back inside. He did exactly what he set out to do. Chalk one up in the victory column. It wasn't long before Dan's neighbor started going to the mailbox without his morning coffee, and shortly after that he'd walk to the light pole up the road. Within a few weeks, he was walking to the stop sign down the block. You can see where the story is going, right? Within months, he was actively jogging around the neighborhood feeling great.

Most people overlook the importance of winning when it comes to building confidence—but not Dan Russell. Dan knew that at the end of the day, confidence trumps just about everything else and to be confident, you need to know how to win. Simple as that. And that neighbor? Now he's in great shape, and those feelings of being powerless to change his life are a distant memory.

What was the first thing you did this morning? What about the hour before you went to bed last night? What happened the last time you became frustrated? Your reaction to life's challenges often doesn't involve careful consideration or divine inspiration. Habit is the driving force behind much of what you do. Without conscious thought, habits kick in and relieve you of having to think. Your habits influence how you feel, what you experience, and, ultimately, who you become. Without realizing it, Dan's advice helped his neighbor form new positive habits and build confidence in the process.

Think about the time you spend driving your car, successfully navigating hundreds of obstacles with little conscious thought. The well-conditioned habit of driving delivers you safely home. The same goes for riding a bike. Initially, intense concentration and effort were required not to crash, but after a short time conquering your neighborhood was a breeze. We rely on habits to manage the monumental volume of information and decisions we're bombarded with throughout the day. But depending on the quality of our habits, they lift us up or tear us down.

Some habits anchor quickly, while others take longer. Did you know a physiological addiction to nicotine takes 1 to 2 years to develop? Smokers must invest time overcoming the painful sensation of inhaling smoke. Thankfully, when making healthy additions to your life, it often only takes a few weeks to settle into a new routine—as long as these new activities fit your lifestyle and personal preferences.

Creating new, empowering habits and breaking old, unwanted patterns requires effort. Self-reflection is necessary to gain insight into the habits that are holding you back and what behaviors are needed to achieve your goals. Here's a good place to start.

1. **Get clear on what you would like to improve.** Many people have no problem telling you everything they don't want, but struggle to identify what they truly desire. Your brain needs a target to focus on. Unique goals require different strategies, so write down your vision for the future or, at the very least, say it out loud. The more specific you are, the more effective you'll be at finding your way.

2. **What habits have created your current situation?** We all run patterns, made up of habits that we have subconsciously developed over the years. Successful coaches study opponents, looking at their patterns and natural tendencies. This is valuable information when creating a game plan for an upcoming game or match. Adopt the role of coach and identify your own patterns. What happens around the time you indulge in food that contributes to your weight problem?

When you become frustrated or stressed what behaviors do you naturally revert to? Some will be valuable and others detrimental. Strengthen the positive habits you already possess and start eliminating the harmful patterns one by one.

3. **What new habits do you need to acquire?** Becoming an evolved version of yourself is necessary if lasting change is going to stick. Imagine the lifestyle required to live your goals. What foods are prioritized? How does exercise fit into a daily routine? How will you manage stress? Are you willing to live your life under these conditions? If the answer is no, you need to come up with a different, more compelling plan.

## HABIT FORMATION

In the early 1990s, researchers at MIT discovered that at the core of every habit is a neurological loop comprising three distinct components: a cue or trigger, a routine, and a reward. To form a new habit, you must find a way to break this loop and replace old, destructive behaviors with more empowering alternatives.

The birth of a habit begins the moment you decide to take action, and with enough repetition any behavior, good or bad, can become automatic. As new thoughts or behaviors are repeated, connections between the neurons in your brain begin to change. Since our brains are as unique as fingerprints, we all have slightly different responses. A habit that takes you a week to develop may take a friend much longer. But researchers who study habit formation have demonstrated that physical changes in the brain can occur in as little as one week. Here's a step-by-step approach to break down old, unhealthy patterns and the habits that feed them and replace them with empowering alternatives.

### Identify the Pattern

The first step in the process involves learning to recognize your patterns. Since your goal is to lose weight, examine your routines around eating. Maybe you have developed the habit of snacking throughout the day, or you regularly pull into a drive-thru on your way home from work. Pay close attention to the choices you make because it's often only two or three patterns that have contributed to much of your weight gain. Once these are identified, they become much easier to manage.

## Discover the Trigger

When it comes to unhealthy eating, what sets you off? Do you start focusing on everything that needs to get done and end up feeling stressed as a result? When you are bored, do you use food as a distraction? Or has eating become a hobby you share with friends? Almost every cue or trigger fits into one of the following five categories.

1. **Location:** If you want to quit drinking alcohol but continue to hang out with your old drinking buddies at the pub, your chance of success diminishes.

2. **Time:** Are you disciplined with your diet throughout the day but break down late at night? Are you a seasonal binge eater? It's easier to create a solution to overcome temptation during specific times of the day if you identify exactly when the problem arises.

3. **Emotional state:** Negative habits are often linked to specific emotional states. Do you find yourself reaching for a cigarette during a stressful moment? When you have a disagreement with a significant other or when your boss is being demanding at work, pay close attention to your reactions. Even small, mundane frustrations—such as someone cutting you off in traffic—can affect your emotional state, leading to unhealthy decisions.

4. **Other people:** There are people who bring out the best in us, and others who . . . don't. Spending time with certain people leads us to eat poorly, exercise harder, and everything in between those two extremes. Connect with those who compel you to become a better version of yourself.

5. **Actions:** Some habits are triggered by specific actions, such as grabbing a beer and a snack before you sit on the couch. Do you even remember opening that bag of chips? Are you even hungry?

## Identify the Rewards

All habits have rewards attached to them, even the destructive ones. Otherwise, why would you invest the time repeating a behavior long enough for it to become an automatic response? If you find yourself repeating a pattern over and over, it's because you're receiving some form of benefit. It may be anything from stress release to connecting with loved ones to feeling significant. It's important to find out what that benefit is so you can still meet your emotional needs in a way that doesn't negatively impact your health. Touching a hot stove as a child didn't provide much benefit, so it never became a habit. Smoking or drinking, even though they both lead to an early death, provide benefits. Stress relief or connection to others—whatever the reward, it's there.

## Break the Cycle

Breaking the cycle sounds dramatic, but it's not all that complicated. You just have to pay attention to the patterns you habitually run. When the urge to repeat an old habit surfaces, immediately take action in another direction. If you have the habit of checking to see if everything is okay in the refrigerator 10 times a day, the moment you catch yourself opening the door of the fridge, go for a walk around the block instead.

When Ryan's daughter was 8, she started using the word "like" way too much, but the frequency dropped considerably when she had to do five pushups every time it was used inappropriately. When you interrupt a pattern, the established neurological sequence linked to a specific behavior becomes scrambled and harder to run.

## Replace with a New Behavior

Trying to eliminate unwanted habits is a challenge if you don't replace them with new behaviors that meet the emotional needs the old habit was servicing. If you get bored during the day and eating snack foods is how you distract yourself, you'll need a new behavior that will also keep you from feeling bored—hopefully one that will not also make you overeat. If losing your temper is your way of releasing stress, you must find an alternative that provides these benefits that doesn't tear down your relationships. When you interrupt an old pattern and introduce a healthy alternative that meets your emotional needs, you'll have stopped the negative cycle. Try doing five pushups every time you reach for a snack. We'd be willing to bet that after the 7 seconds it takes to complete those pushups, you'll be rethinking your snack plans. Physical movement provides endless pattern-breaking opportunities; a walk around the block, 20 squats, or a sprint up the stairs are all effective.

## Condition the New Behavior

Once you have chosen a more empowering option, you must make sure it sticks. This is accomplished by conditioning and involves repeating the new behavior until it becomes natural. In athletics this is called drilling, and it's the most effective way to learn any new technique. Here's how it works. Under low stress, you repeat a new movement pattern over and over, paying attention to every detail, until you can perform the technique without conscious thought under the stress of competition.

When conditioning new behaviors, the first several weeks require the most focus and discipline, but you will be surprised by how quickly new habits start to feel less foreign. Remain consistent and when you mess up, immediately correct yourself, leaving out the negative self-talk. Compelling goals provide the motivation needed to stay focused long enough for new patterns to become automatic. Without a strategy or specific plan, you will inevitably revert to old patterns. Good habits take effort to develop, but you'll have no trouble living with the results. Bad habits come easy, but you won't like the consequences.

At the beginning of each year, many people make New Year's resolutions. These often involve eliminating unwanted behaviors we know we should change but haven't found a way to do so. But how many people actually stick to those resolutions? Can you name one New Year's resolution that you've successfully integrated into your life? This is a prime example of trying to change a habit without following the steps outlined above. Every habit you've created has served a purpose and somehow meets specific emotional needs. Eliminating a bad habit without replacing it with something else that meets the same needs is a recipe for failure. In 2012, the *Journal of the American Medical Association* published a study that showed people who elected to have gastric bypass surgery were at a higher risk for developing an addiction to alcohol afterward. Reducing the size of the stomach didn't eliminate the emotional needs overeating provided, so alcohol was substituted for food. Out of the pot and into the fire. There is the pain of discipline and the pain of regret. You must pick one. Where would you rather suffer?

## Pavlov's Dogs

If you've ever taken a psychology class, you may remember Ivan Pavlov, a Russian physiologist who, in the 1890s, studied why dogs salivate before being fed. Dogs don't have to learn how to salivate; it's innate. Behaviorists call this an unconditioned response. Food (the stimulus) triggered an unconditioned response: excess saliva.

After some time in the lab, Pavlov recognized that the dogs began to salivate when his lab assistant, who fed them, walked into the room. It didn't matter whether he was carrying a bowl of food. Since the dogs did not salivate at the sight of the lab assistant before these experiments began, Pavlov understood that the dogs must have learned this association.

Pavlov decided to explore this phenomenon further and wondered if he could cause this response with a completely unrelated stimulus. So he began a new experiment. This

## HABIT FORMATION IN ACTION

**One day my wife gently hinted that I could be doing more around the house to help out, and she was right.** Without saying anything, I decided I would start with the dishes. If there was a dish in the sink, no matter what I was doing, I would stop to wash it, dry it, and put it away. This may not seem like much on the surface, but it went a long way with her. I was a little surprised to discover that most of the time this took less than one minute. In addition to making my wife happier, there was also a small sense of accomplishment. I liked it. Within a week, washing the dishes the moment I noticed them sitting in the sink seemed normal. After a month, I didn't ever think about it. If there was a dirty dish, I would wash it. The times when a hint of procrastination set in, I refused to acknowledge it. Robbing procrastination of its power was easy because I had trained myself to take action at the sight of a dish in the sink. In addition to a cleaner house, I was given the additional reward of a happier wife. Never underestimate the power of a happy woman.

**If doing the dishes added an extra 10 minutes of work to my day, I would be surprised.** So once I had that mastered that task, I quietly looked for more opportunities to help out. I found the laundry. Since my approach with the dishes worked so well, I repeated the process. If I walked by the washer and noticed a finished load, I would throw it in the dryer. This never takes longer than 15 seconds. If there was a dry load sitting in the dryer, I'd fold it. This rarely took more than 5 minutes. Although the effort required was minimal, it made a dramatic difference in how our days went. Even if we put aside the improved family dynamics, the conscious act of doing the dishes and the laundry helped defeat procrastination in other areas. The 2 years following these changes were the most productive and lucrative of my entire life.

time, prior to the dogs being fed, Pavlov would ring a bell. He kept repeating this pattern: ringing the bell, then feeding the dogs. He discovered it didn't take long for the dogs to salivate the moment they heard the bell ring.

This trick is not just a dog phenomenon. Do you remember the frenzy a neighborhood ice cream truck would create on a hot summer day when you were a kid? The music, heard blocks away, would cause kids to race home and beg their parents for money to buy a Fudgsicle. It happens with chickens as well. Years ago, Ryan had neighbors that kept chickens in their backyard, and he'd occasionally feed them table scraps over the fence. Before long, whenever he pulled into his driveway, eight chickens would come running up to greet him. Dogs, chickens, or humans, we're making associations all the time—some good, others not so good. But these stories illustrate the power that reward has on our habits.

---

UFC fighter Ed Herman has been a training partner and teammate of mine for as long as I can remember. When Ed fought Tim Boetsch in the UFC, he put on a hell of a performance and was rewarded by the UFC with a bonus, above and beyond what they were contractually obligated to pay. In Ed's case, it was an additional $50,000. He was set for the year—time to party. But then Ed sustained a knee injury that required surgery. Due to inactivity, his weight went up to 225 pounds and he was so out of shape he could barely breathe when his heart rate went above 140 beats per minute.

Around this time, I was scheduled to fight Michael Bisping and I needed Ed as a training partner. But no matter how many times I called him, he told me, "I can't do it." So the next time I saw him, I threw my arm around him. "Okay," I said. "Here's what you're going to do. Next week, starting on Monday, come to practice at 6:30 p.m. You're not working out, so come dressed in street clothes and watch practice." I needed to get him used to coming back to the gym without any pressure. The following week I told him, "This week, you're going to come in every day at 6:30 p.m., complete the warmup and you're done. No matter how you feel, you're done after the warmup." At the start of the third week I asked him to complete the warmup and technical drilling portion of the workouts. It wasn't until week 4 that live sparring was included in his training. Ed followed my advice and before long was back to training with full intensity.

Creating anything worthwhile in life is a process, including healthy habits. We all have habits at various stages of development, including new behaviors or thought patterns that require lots of focus to implement and others that don't require much effort anymore. This process continues throughout life. A clear vision of what's important helps develop the discipline needed to make consistent effort to anchor new behaviors.

## THE 12 ESSENTIAL NUTRITION HABITS

If you're looking for some inspiration, here's a list of 12 habits that will pull you in the direction of your four-pack goal.

### Habit 1: Eat Slowly

Our fast food culture has created an army of speed-eaters. Leave that for Joey Chestnut and put the fork down. This habit has nothing to do with *what* you're eating, but it can have a dramatic impact on *how much* you're eating. Why? There's a delay between when the food reaches your stomach and when your brain realizes you're full. Slowing down while you eat helps you become aware of your hunger and other appetite cues. If it takes 15 to 20 minutes to finish your meal, then you're doing well.

Eating meals with others is always a good idea, as you'll naturally break up your eating with conversation. Your relationships will benefit, you'll eat less, and enjoy your food more. If you're always on the go and 20 minutes per meal is out of the question, then lower your expectations. Take five minutes instead of two. Anything extra will help—just get something in your win column.

### Habit 2: Stop Eating at 80 Percent Full

This takes some discipline as well, especially if you're a fast eater or let yourself get overly hungry by waiting long periods of time between meals. Waiting for your brain to catch up with your stomach can feel like eternity. Eating slowly (Habit 1) makes it easier to stop when you've had enough to eat.

Here's a timeline of how you should feel after eating.

- **Immediately after:** You're still craving a little more–if there's food left on the table, you'll want to eat it. Resist the urge and wait a few minutes. Walk out of the kitchen and around the block if need be.
- **One hour after eating:** You're no longer thinking about food. If you're craving something, it's an emotional response and food can't fix that problem.
- **Two hours later:** You may find yourself thinking about your next meal. You could eat, but the urge is not that strong. You'll be able to continue going about your day without distraction. Drink two glasses of water.
- **Three hours later:** Okay, it's almost time to eat, but your hunger isn't making you too grumpy. Thankfully, you've planned your day, and a balanced meal is not far away. If you're not hungry at this point, chances are you ate too much at your last meal.
- **Four hours later:** You have one priority, and that is to eat. Now.

## Habit 3: Eat Protein-Dense Foods with Each Meal

Eating protein, 20 to 30 grams with each meal, stimulates your metabolism, improves muscle mass, and reduces body fat. Remember from our discussion of portion size in Chapter 4: A good gauge is to use the size of your palm as a visual reference for an adequate portion size. Meaning if a piece of wild salmon is about the same size as your palm, you're looking good.

## Habit 4: Eat Vegetables at Every Meal

Not only are vegetables low in calories and high in fiber, they are also loaded with micronutrients essential for cellular health. The alkaline effect of vegetables helps offset the acidic nature of protein and grains while feeding the healthy colony of bacteria in your gut. So eat your veggies, often and in whatever form you can.

We're also big on the benefits of juicing green vegetables such as cucumber, celery, spinach, kale, parsley, and chard. We have used fresh veggie juices for enhanced nutrition during strenuous training and weight cutting for years. Green juices are a healthy way to increase your water intake and are loaded with nutrition. Naturally low in sugar, they also

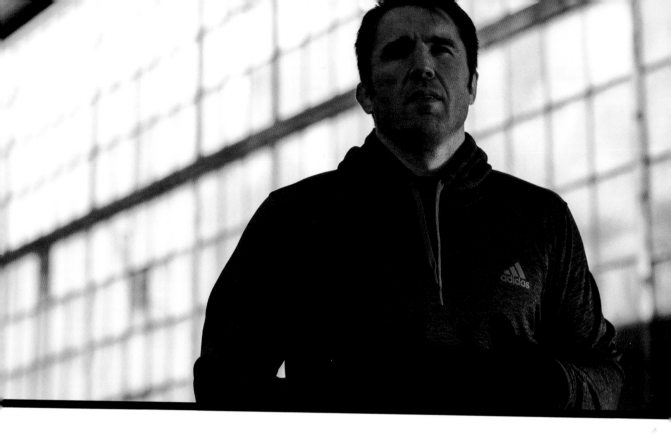

work well as an appetite suppressant. While there are many approaches to dieting, it's rare to find a popular diet that doesn't recommend eating vegetables.

## Habit 5: Enjoy Carbohydrates

Forget no carb, forget high carb—you need a balanced, healthy approach to carbs to keep you going. Carbs make meals more satisfying. They taste good, and the ones we recommend are high in fiber. Just avoid anything starchy and white (potatoes, rice, sugar, or anything processed). Healthy carbs are easy to come by: Non-starchy vegetables, lentils, beans, peas, and cauliflower are all excellent choices.

## Habit 6: Eat Similar Meals

A few go-to meals make the process of healthy eating much easier. This approach requires less thought, it's easier to measure portion size, and if you know you enjoy the food, you'll have a better chance of following through. If you get bored, you can always spice things up or use different condiments for a change in flavor.

## Habit 7: Drink Water, Not Sugar Water

If you're looking for one thing to change in your diet, start here. Fruit juice-based drinks and sodas are loaded with sugar and calories, and expose you to a number of health risks from tooth decay to weight gain. Replacing them with water or herbal teas is not difficult to do and is the easiest way to improve your diet. Let's add diet soda here as well, even though it's technically low in sugar. Recent research indicates that consumption of diet soda may triple the risk of stroke and dementia.

## Habit 8: Increase Lean Body Mass

Your weight loss will primarily come from changes in your diet, not exercise. Still, building lean body mass (a.k.a. muscle) is an integral part of the fat-loss equation. Muscle tissue increases your metabolism and naturally burns more calories. Plus, you'll look, feel, and move better. No matter what age you are, your muscles will respond if you challenge them. If you're out of shape, don't rush this process—start slow and build up. As your diet improves and your weight comes down, your energy will increase. Most people overestimate what they can do in a month and underestimate what they can achieve in a year. In 12 months, you can radically transform your body.

## Habit 9: Decrease Inflammation

Inflammation is a natural response the body uses to protect itself. For acute injuries, inflammation is beneficial and stimulates the healing process. Chronic inflammation, on the other hand, is dangerous and contributes to an increased risk of diseases such as diabetes, heart disease, and obesity. Many people suffer from chronic, low-grade inflammation, and a sedentary lifestyle, lack of sleep, stress, and poor diet all contribute to the problem.

Eliminating the worst offenders—sugar, processed carbs, trans fats, processed meat, and alcohol—will also have a major impact on reducing inflammation. Sound familiar? These foods keep coming up over and over as red flags. Thankfully, inflammation is pretty easy to correct, and the foundation foods of this plan—beans, fish, nuts, seeds, and veggies—will help balance your system.

## Habit 10: Manage Cravings

Cravings happen to everyone. Pretending you're never going to eat a piece of fried chicken again is not entirely reasonable, so plan to eat your favorite foods with a weekly System Reset meal. If your cravings seem out of control or are stubbornly persistent, try adding more protein to your diet. Protein has been shown to reduce cravings. Also, make sure you're properly hydrated and eating enough. Remember, you shouldn't be hungry an hour after a meal. If you are, take a deep breath and reel those emotions back in.

## Habit 11: Learn Portion Size

As we mentioned previously, counting calories is tough, but having several go-to meals makes staying on track much easier. A meal should consist of:

- 2 palm-size portions of protein
- 1 palm-size serving of complex carbohydrates
- 2 handfuls of vegetables
- 1 tablespoon of oil

This formula is easy for anyone to remember and works while eating at home or dining out. Remember, a serving size is the amount of food indicated on a food label; a portion is how much food you choose to eat at one time. Pay attention to how the portions you eat relate to the serving size noted on the food label when calculating the nutritional value of your meal. When you dine out, don't let the chef determine how much you'll eat.

## Habit 12: Have a Plan for When Things Fall Apart

There will rarely be a week that passes in which everything goes to plan. Life offers constant opportunities to learn to adapt when the unexpected comes your way. On occasion, you'll eat something unhealthy or find yourself out of time when you were planning

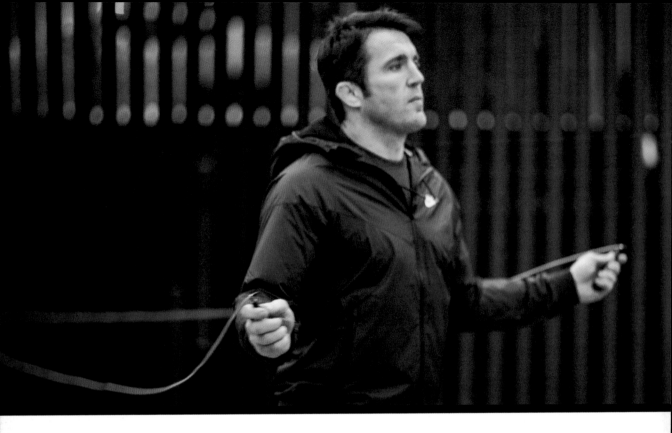

to work out. Anticipate these challenges and be ready for them. Don't be one of those people who throw everything away because one or two things didn't go as planned. Eliminate negative thinking and instead devise a plan for what you'll do when things go awry.

So there you have it: 12 excellent habits that you can take on to make a lasting change in both how you eat and how you feel. But remember, small steps. Don't feel obligated to take on all 12 at once. Experiment and see what works best for you.

# 9
# MEAL PLAN PREPARATION

**W**E CAN'T STRESS THIS ENOUGH–DESPITE WHAT THE LATEST INFOMERCIAL promises, you cannot exercise your way to a four-pack. Or any size pack, for that matter. So make each meal count and remember: Consistency delivers results and the single best way to remain consistent is to prepare. If you're stocked up on Four-Pack foods and you make the effort to prep meals in advance, you're 80 percent of the way there. Planning creates flexibility, which makes managing your meals virtually painless. And with an endless variety of dishes that taste great and are good for you, there's no excuse not to eat well.

## UPGRADES AND SUBSTITUTIONS

When creating your meal plans, look for ways to make small changes that will, over time, lead to significant results. These upgrades and substitutions shave calories and increase the nutritional benefits of the foods you consume.

### Upgrades

Adding a few teaspoons of hempseed, chia seeds, or flaxseed to a smoothie delivers a healthy dose of essential omega-3 oils. Switching from refined vegetable oil to one like Apollo Olive Oil eliminates unhealthy processed fats. We use kombucha tea to help control cravings, and it may improve digestion and overall gut health. There are lots of opportunities to increase the quality of your meals that require very little effort or expense.

### Substitutions

Substituting healthier food options can make dietary changes more manageable. For example, give Banza pasta a try–this pasta substitute made from chickpeas is an alternative for those who love a plate of pasta. Depending on how you drink your coffee, learning to appreciate it unsweetened (or without cream) can eliminate a significant number of calories. Using a teaspoon of olive oil on your salad instead of a tablespoon saves 80 calories. This may not seem like much, but that's a 4 percent calorie reduction over the course of the day and you most likely won't notice the difference. Imagine the benefits if you found five or six ways to cut calories and improve the health properties of the food you eat daily. Over the course of a month, those changes would add up and you wouldn't feel like you've sacrificed much. It just requires paying attention, so examine your diet and look for opportunities to make these small changes.

The ideal Four-Pack meal should follow these basic guidelines.

- Half your plate is filled with vegetables.
- Eat a handful of slow-digesting carbohydrates.
- Include a palm-size portion of protein with each meal.
- Include healthy fats too–about a tablespoon.

## SHOPPING LIST

| | | | |
|---|---|---|---|
| **PROTEIN** | Wild salmon | **STARCHES** | Lentils |
| | Wild halibut | | Garbanzo beans |
| | Omega/free-range eggs | | Black beans |
| | Organic poultry | | Great northern beans |
| | Grass-raised lamb | | Pinto beans |
| | Grass-raised beef | | Quinoa |
| **VEGETABLES** | Broccoli | | Sprouted breads |
| | Cauliflower | | Yams |
| | Spinach | | Squash |
| | Chard | **FATS/OILS** | Olive oil |
| | Kale | | Ghee |
| | Green/red/yellow peppers | | Coconut oil |
| | Artichoke | | Fish oil supplement |
| | Brussels sprouts | **FRUIT** | Lemons |
| | Zucchini | | Limes |
| | Parsley | | Grapefruit |
| | Arugula | | Blueberries |
| | Cilantro | | Blackberries |
| | Tomatoes | | |
| | Cabbage | | |
| | Sprouts | | |

## SAMPLE DAILY MEAL PLAN—4 MEALS

| QTY | MEASURE | DESCRIPTION | PROTEIN (GM) | CARBS (GM) | FATS (GM) | CALORIES |
|---|---|---|---|---|---|---|
| **Meal 1** | | | | | | |
| 1.00 | slice | Sprouted Grain Bread | 4.00 | 15.00 | 0.50 | 80.00 |
| 3.00 | large | Eggs | 18.00 | 0.00 | 15.00 | 210.00 |
| 6.00 | ounces | Garbanzo Beans | 15.00 | 46.65 | 4.35 | 276.00 |
| 1.00 | tablespoon | Extra Virgin Olive Oil | 0.00 | 0.00 | 14.00 | 120.00 |
| 2.00 | 1 cup | Spinach | 1.72 | 2.18 | 0.23 | 13.80 |
| **Totals:** | | | 38.72 | 68.83 | 34.08 | 699.80 |
| **Meal 2** | | | | | | |
| 1.00 | each | Banana | 1.20 | 26.70 | 0.60 | 105.00 |
| 1.00 | scoop | Protein Powder | 20.95 | 19.33 | 1.57 | 178.20 |
| 6.00 | ounces | Coffee | 0.20 | 0.70 | 0.00 | 6.00 |
| 0.50 | 1 oz | Chia Seeds | 2.34 | 5.97 | 4.36 | 68.89 |
| 1.00 | 1 cup | Unsweetened almond milk | 6.37 | 9.36 | 2.07 | 82.62 |
| **Totals:** | | | 31.06 | 62.06 | 8.59 | 440.71 |
| **Meal 3** | | | | | | |
| 2.00 | 0.5 cup | Arugula | 0.52 | 0.73 | 0.13 | 5.00 |
| 0.50 | 1 fruit, without skin and seed | Avocados | 1.33 | 5.88 | 10.48 | 113.56 |
| 6.00 | ounces | Chicken Breast | 39.00 | 0.00 | 2.40 | 186.00 |
| 0.50 | tablespoon | Extra Virgin Olive Oil | 0.00 | 0.00 | 7.00 | 60.00 |
| 1.00 | 1 cup | Quinoa | 8.14 | 39.41 | 3.55 | 222.00 |
| **Totals:** | | | 48.99 | 46.01 | 23.56 | 586.56 |
| **Meal 4** | | | | | | |
| 1.00 | tablespoon | Butter or Ghee | 0.12 | 0.01 | 11.52 | 101.81 |
| 2.00 | 3 oz | Halibut | 38.32 | 0.00 | 2.74 | 188.70 |
| 1.00 | 1 cup | Lentils | 17.86 | 39.86 | 0.75 | 229.68 |
| 2.00 | 1 cup | Spinach | 1.72 | 2.18 | 0.23 | 13.80 |
| 1.00 | 1 medium (2" dia, 5" long, raw) | Sweet Potato | 2.29 | 23.61 | 0.117 | 102.60 |
| **Totals:** | | | 60.31 | 65.65 | 15.41 | 636.59 |
| **Totals for Day:** | | | 179.07 | 237.55 | 81.65 | 2363.66 |
| % of Total Calories: | | | 29.83 | 39.57 | 30.60 | |

## SAMPLE DAILY MEAL PLAN—5 MEALS

| QTY | MEASURE | DESCRIPTION | PROTEIN (GM) | CARBS (GM) | FATS (GM) | CALORIES |
|---|---|---|---|---|---|---|
| *Meal 1* | | | | | | |
| 3.00 | large | Eggs | 18.00 | 0.00 | 15.00 | 210.00 |
| 6.00 | ounces | Garbanzo Beans | 15.00 | 46.65 | 4.35 | 276.00 |
| 1.00 | tablespoon | Extra Virgin Olive Oil | 0.00 | 0.00 | 14.00 | 120.00 |
| 1.00 | 1 cup | Spinach | 0.86 | 1.09 | 0.12 | 6.90 |
| Totals: | | | 33.86 | 47.74 | 33.47 | 612.90 |
| *Meal 2* | | | | | | |
| 1.00 | 1 scoop | Protein Powder | 20.95 | 19.33 | 1.57 | 178.20 |
| 6.00 | ounces | Coffee | 0.20 | 0.70 | 0.00 | 6.00 |
| 1.00 | 1 cup | Unsweetened almond milk | 6.37 | 9.36 | 2.07 | 82.62 |
| Totals: | | | 27.52 | 29.39 | 3.64 | 266.82 |
| *Meal 3* | | | | | | |
| 2.00 | 0.5 cup | Arugula | 0.52 | 0.73 | 0.13 | 5.00 |
| 1.00 | 1 fruit, without skin and seed | Avocado | 2.67 | 11.75 | 20.96 | 227.12 |
| 6.00 | ounces | Chicken Breast | 39.00 | 0.00 | 2.40 | 186.00 |
| 1.00 | 1 cup | Quinoa | 8.14 | 39.41 | 3.55 | 222.00 |
| Totals: | | | 50.32 | 51.89 | 27.04 | 640.12 |
| *Meal 4* | | | | | | |
| 1.00 | each | Banana | 1.20 | 26.70 | 0.60 | 105.00 |
| 5.00 | ounces | Greek Yogurt (nonfat) | 10.00 | 5.00 | 0.00 | 75.00 |
| 0.19 | 1 oz | Chia Seeds | 0.89 | 2.27 | 1.66 | 26.18 |
| 1.00 | 1 teaspoon, ground | Flaxseeds | 0.46 | 0.72 | 1.05 | 13.35 |
| Totals: | | | 12.55 | 34.69 | 3.31 | 219.53 |
| *Meal 5* | | | | | | |
| 2.00 | slice | Sprouted Grain Bread | 8.00 | 30.00 | 1.00 | 160.00 |
| 2.00 | 3 oz | Halibut | 38.32 | 0.00 | 2.74 | 188.70 |
| 0.75 | 1 cup | Lentils | 13.39 | 29.89 | 0.56 | 172.26 |
| 2.00 | 1 cup | Spinach | 1.72 | 2.18 | 0.23 | 13.80 |
| Totals: | | | 61.43 | 62.07 | 4.54 | 534.76 |
| Totals for Day: | | | 185.68 | 225.78 | 71.99 | 2274.13 |
| % of Total Calories: | | | 32.38 | 39.37 | 28.25 | |

## SAMPLE DAILY MEAL PLAN—6 MEALS

| QTY | MEASURE | DESCRIPTION | PROTEIN (GM) | CARBS (GM) | FATS (GM) | CALORIES |
|---|---|---|---|---|---|---|
| Meal 1 | | | | | | |
| 3.00 | large | Eggs | 18.00 | 0.00 | 15.00 | 210.00 |
| 5.00 | ounces | Garbanzo Beans | 12.50 | 38.88 | 3.62 | 230.00 |
| 1.00 | tablespoon | Extra Virgin Olive Oil | 0.00 | 0.00 | 14.00 | 120.00 |
| 1.00 | 1 cup | Spinach | 0.86 | 1.09 | 0.12 | 6.90 |
| Totals: | | | 31.36 | 39.96 | 32.74 | 566.90 |
| Meal 2 | | | | | | |
| 1.00 | scoop | Protein Powder | 20.95 | 19.33 | 1.57 | 178.20 |
| 6.00 | ounces | Coffee | 0.20 | 0.70 | 0.00 | 6.00 |
| 1.00 | 1 cup | Unsweetened Almond Milk | 6.37 | 9.36 | 2.07 | 82.62 |
| Totals: | | | 27.52 | 29.39 | 3.64 | 266.82 |
| Meal 3 | | | | | | |
| 2.00 | 0.5 cup | Arugula | 0.52 | 0.73 | 0.13 | 5.00 |
| 0.50 | 1 fruit, without skin and seed | Avocados | 1.33 | 5.88 | 10.48 | 113.56 |
| 6.00 | ounces | Chicken Breast | 39.00 | 0.00 | 2.40 | 186.00 |
| 1.00 | 1 cup | Quinoa | 8.14 | 39.41 | 3.55 | 222.00 |
| Totals: | | | 48.99 | 46.01 | 16.56 | 526.56 |
| Meal 4 | | | | | | |
| 1.00 | each | Banana | 1.20 | 26.70 | 0.60 | 105.00 |
| 5.00 | ounces | Greek Yogurt (nonfat) | 10.00 | 5.00 | 0.00 | 75.00 |
| 0.19 | 1 oz | Chia Seeds | 0.89 | 2.27 | 1.66 | 26.18 |
| 1.00 | 1 teaspoon, ground | Flaxseeds | 0.46 | 0.72 | 1.05 | 13.35 |
| Totals: | | | 12.55 | 34.69 | 3.31 | 219.53 |
| Meal 5 | | | | | | |
| 2.00 | slice | Sprouted Grain Bread | 8.00 | 30.00 | 1.00 | 160.00 |
| 2.00 | 3 oz | Halibut | 38.32 | 0.00 | 2.74 | 188.70 |
| 0.75 | 1 cup | Lentils | 13.39 | 29.89 | 0.56 | 172.26 |
| 2.00 | 1 cup | Spinach | 1.72 | 2.18 | 0.23 | 13.80 |
| Totals: | | | 61.43 | 62.07 | 4.54 | 534.76 |
| Meal 6 | | | | | | |
| 2.00 | tablespoon | Almond butter | 4.00 | 6.00 | 18.00 | 202.00 |
| 2.00 | each | Celery | 1.00 | 4.00 | 0.00 | 20.00 |
| 1.00 | 1 miniature box (.5 oz) | Raisins | 0.43 | 11.09 | 0.06 | 41.86 |
| Totals: | | | 5.43 | 21.09 | 18.06 | 263.86 |
| Totals for Day: | | | 187.27 | 233.21 | 78.85 | 2378.43 |
| % of Total Calories | | | 31.32 | 39.01 | 29.67 | |

# RECESPES
# SMOOTHIES

Smoothies are an easy way to create a nutritious meal or snack in minutes. Adding protein supplements, essential fatty acids, or even leafy greens such as spinach can increase a smoothie's nutritional value. A high-powered blender like a Vitamix is an essential kitchen appliance that makes exceptional smoothies and will last for many years. The Ninja is a less expensive option that also works great.

## COLD BREW PROTEIN
# SMOOTHIE

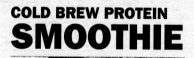

**PREP TIME: 5 MINUTES**
**SERVINGS: 1**

In the past year or so, we have become fans of cold brew coffee. Coffee is loaded with antioxidants, and the simple process of cold brewing creates a strong coffee concentrate that's less acidic than traditional brewing methods. The ratio (4:1) is four parts water to one part coarse ground coffee. This strong concentrate can be diluted with water or milk. Unsweetened almond milk, found at most grocery stores, is an excellent, healthy choice and pairs well with the coffee flavor. Check the label of your protein powder for sugar content. Only add a sweetener if necessary. Alternatively, half a frozen banana will add sugar in a natural form.

| | |
|---|---|
| 1 | scoop chocolate protein powder |
| ³/₄ | cup cold brew coffee |
| ³/₄ | cup unsweetened almond milk |
| 1 | tablespoon nut butter* (optional) |
| | Ice (optional) |

Place all ingredients in the blender for 30 seconds.

•You can choose any nut butter, keeping in mind that this will increase the calorie count of your smoothie.

## MATCHA GREEN TEA
# SMOOTHIE

**PREP TIME: 5 MINUTES**
**SERVINGS: 1**

| | |
|---|---|
| 12 | ounces unsweetened almond milk |
| 1 | frozen banana |
| ½ | cup ice |
| 2 | tablespoons protein powder |
| 2 | teaspoons matcha green tea powder |
| 1 | teaspoon agave nectar (optional) |

Matcha powder is the powdered whole green tea leaf that has been used in Japan for 900 years. Since you consume the entire leaf when you drink matcha, you receive small amounts of vitamins and minerals as well as polyphenols such as EGCG, which has been shown to boost metabolism and slow or halt the growth of cancer cells.

Place all ingredients in the blender for 30 seconds.

## POWER GREEN
# SMOOTHIE

**PREP TIME: 5 MINUTES**
**SERVINGS: 1**

| | |
|---|---|
| 1 | cup kale |
| 1 | cup spinach leaves |
| 1 | frozen banana (slice before freezing) |
| ½ | green apple |
| 1 | tablespoon flaxseed |
| ½ | cup ice |
| ½ | cup water |
| 2 | tablespoons protein powder (optional) |

Adding vegetables to smoothies is one of the best ways to consume more of these essential foods. You always have the option of adding a scoop or two of protein powder if you're using a smoothie for a meal replacement and would like to increase the nutritional content. Experiment with your own version of this recipe to suit your taste.

Place all ingredients in the blender for 30 seconds.

# AVOCADO GREEN
# SMOOTHIE

**PREP TIME: 5 MINUTES**
**SERVINGS: 2**

Adding an avocado to a smoothie may sound strange, but it works. In addition to supplying healthy fats, avocado is high in fiber and adds a rich creaminess to this smoothie. A scoop of protein powder works here as well if you are looking to add more protein to your diet. This is an easy recipe to customize. A banana will produce a smoother final product that is a bit sweeter. You can easily add nutritional supplements like essential fatty acids as well.

²/₃   cup unsweetened almond milk

2     large handfuls spinach leaves or kale, or both

¹/₂   frozen banana (slice before freezing)

¹/₂   avocado, sliced

1     scoop protein powder

1     cup ice

1     tablespoon flaxseed or essential fatty acids supplement (optional)

Place all ingredients in the blender for 30 seconds.

# BLUEBERRY
# BOWL

**PREP TIME: 3 MINUTES**
**SERVINGS: 1**

Dark berries such as blueberries are naturally low in sugar, high in fiber, and loaded with antioxidants. A blueberry bowl is a great snack or dessert that is ready in minutes. If you need a snack before going to bed, try this recipe to take the edge off.

1     cup blueberries

1     cup unsweetened almond milk

1     handful chopped raw nuts (almonds or cashews)

1     frozen banana (slice before freezing; optional)

1     tablespoon flaxseed (optional)

2     tablespoons protein powder, preferably unflavored (optional)

1     teaspoon essential oil supplement (optional)

Place all ingredients in the blender for 30 seconds. Another option is to combine the ingredients in a bowl and eat with a spoon. In this case, use fresh banana and add the chopped nuts on top.

# VEGETABLES

Vegetables are the foundation of any healthy meal. They are nutritious, help promote healthy gut bacteria, and supply high-quality fiber and micronutrients. The key is experimenting to find ways to prepare vegetables that you enjoy eating. Most importantly, prepare vegetables in advance so there are leftovers in the refrigerator to add to every meal.

## POWER GREEN
## SALAD

**PREP TIME: 20 MINUTES**
**SERVINGS: 4**

The secret to eating more vegetables is to have them prepared ahead of time. This salad will keep for a few days and is loaded with nutrition. Kale is an incredibly healthy leafy vegetable and, combined with the lentils and parsley, makes this salad an excellent meal. You could substitute the Parmesan with a half cup of feta cheese, adding it last along with the pepitas. Quinoa can also replace the lentils, although the lentils last a little longer.

| | |
|---|---|
| 3 | cups kale, ribbed and chopped |
| 1/2 | cup chopped parsley |
| 1 | cup cooked green lentils (cook time is 25 minutes) or precooked canned lentils |
| 1 | green apple, diced |
| 1/2 | English cucumber, diced |
| 1/2 | cup shaved Parmesan cheese or nutritional yeast |
| 1/2 | cup toasted pepitas |

### DRESSING

| | |
|---|---|
| 1 | clove garlic |
| 1 | tablespoon honey |
| 1 | tablespoon Dijon mustard |
| | Juice of 1 lemon |
| 1 | tablespoon apple cider vinegar |
| 1/3 | cup extra virgin olive oil |
| | Salt and pepper |

1. In a large bowl, combine the kale, parsley, lentils, apple, cucumber, and Parmesan cheese or nutritional yeast.

2. For the dressing, blitz all the ingredients in a blender until the garlic is smooth. Alternately, you could smash the garlic, chop it fine, mix by hand with the honey and Dijon mustard, and then add the remaining liquids.

3. Pour the dressing on the salad and toss well.

4. Garnish with more Parmesan or nutritional yeast if wanted. Add pepitas last, as the salad is being served. (Pepitas are the only ingredient that will go soggy if mixed in.) Salad lasts well with dressing in fridge for 3 days.

# CAULIFLOWER "STEAKS"

Cauliflower often gets overlooked in the vegetable department. It's loaded with vitamin C and other antioxidants and, like its cousin broccoli, is a member of the cruciferous family of vegetables known for their anti-cancer effects. This recipe is easy to prepare and makes great leftovers. Add two eggs for a quick, healthy breakfast.

**PREP TIME: 3 MINUTES**
**COOK TIME: 35 MINUTES**
**SERVINGS: 6**

1     large head cauliflower

1     tablespoon extra virgin olive oil

     Salt and black cracked pepper

1. Preheat the oven to 350°F.
2. Wash the cauliflower and cut it down the center, making two large halves. Cut ¾-inch slices to get large, full pieces of cauliflower. Make smaller steaks with the outer sections.
3. Place the cauliflower in a large baking dish. Drizzle with olive oil and season with salt and pepper.
4. Place in the oven and cook for 20 minutes.
5. Remove from the oven and turn the pieces over. Cook for another 15 minutes.

# ZUCCHINI SLAW

If you have a food processor, give this a try. Zucchini slaw is light with a great Mediterranean flavor, and will keep for a day or two. If you are preparing larger amounts for the week, keep the dressing separate so the zucchini stays fresh longer.

**PREP TIME: 5 MINUTES**
**COOK TIME: 20 MINUTES**
**SERVINGS: 2**

10     cherry tomatoes

2     teaspoons extra virgin olive oil

     Cracked black pepper

2     large zucchini

4     sprigs parsley

2     teaspoons Pistachio Pesto (page 200)

1. Preheat the oven to 350°F. Line a small baking pan with parchment paper.
2. Rinse the tomatoes and place in the prepared pan. Drizzle with olive oil and top with black pepper. Place in the oven for 15 minutes.
3. Remove the tomatoes from the oven, shake the pan, and place back in the oven for 5 more minutes.
4. Rinse the zucchini and cut them in half. Shred the zucchini in a food processor. Empty into a serving bowl.
5. Add the tomatoes and pesto and toss. Add extra pepper if desired.
6. Garnish with parsley.

## SALT CABBAGE
# SALAD

This salad is a version of a cabbage salad we first had at a Korean BBQ restaurant in Japan. It's easy to make, but you'll need to eat it the same day since the oil and salt will soften the cabbage. This fresh-tasting dish pairs well with chicken, lamb, or beef.

**PREP TIME: 5 MINUTES**
**SERVINGS: 2**

½  head cabbage

½  teaspoon sesame oil

¼  teaspoon chili oil

   Dash soy sauce

⅛  teaspoon Tabasco sauce (optional)

1  teaspoon toasted sesame seeds

   Dash salt

1. Peel off and rinse the cabbage leaves and place them in a medium salad bowl. Break down the larger pieces.

2. Add the remaining ingredients to the bowl and toss together. The oil and salt will wilt the cabbage: simple and delicious.


## BAKED
# ZUCCHINI

Baked zucchini is as simple as a cooked veggie dish can be. They can be prepared whole, sliced in half lengthwise, or chopped into smaller pieces. Seasoned with olive oil, salt, and pepper, this dish can be added to any protein and stores well in the refrigerator for several days.

**PREP TIME: 5 MINUTES**
**COOK TIME: 20 MINUTES**
**SERVINGS: 4**

8  zucchini

1  tablespoon olive oil

   Salt and pepper

1. Preheat the oven to 350°F.

2. Rinse the zucchini and cut to your desired size.

3. Place the zucchini on a baking sheet and coat each piece with olive oil. Bake for 20 minutes.

# HEALTHY STARCHES

Our primary goal with carbohydrates is to rely on the slow-digesting variety. These foods have less impact on blood sugar and are usually high in fiber. Your challenge will be to pay attention to how carbohydrate-rich foods affect you. Some people are more sensitive than others. If this is the case for you, you'll need to dial back starches and increase water-rich vegetables.

# WAFFLES

**PREP TIME: 5 MINUTES**
**COOK TIME: 30 MINUTES**
**SERVINGS: 14**

Who doesn't love waffles? Chael named his dog Danger Waffles. This is one of those recipes to save for a day when you have extra time on your hands. It may take a while to cook the whole batch, but they freeze perfectly and are an excellent, healthy carbohydrate meal that you can grab on your way out the door. They are loaded with healthy ingredients but are not low in calories, so don't eat too many.

| | |
|---|---|
| 6 | cups spelt flour |
| 1/2 | cup rolled oats |
| 1/2 | cup almond meal |
| 1/4 | cup ground chia seeds |
| 1 | teaspoon baking soda |
| 1 | teaspoon baking powder |
| 2 | tablespoons ground flaxseed |
| 1/2 | cup applesauce |
| 2 | teaspoons vanilla extract |
| 1 | liter unsweetened almond milk |
| 1 | tablespoon coconut oil |

1. Preheat a waffle iron.

2. In a large bowl, place the flour, rolled oats, almond meal, ground chia seeds, baking soda, baking powder, and ground flaxseed. Mix together. Gradually add the applesauce, vanilla, almond milk, and coconut oil. If the batter seems too thick, add more almond milk as necessary.

3. Brush some additional coconut oil on the hot waffle iron with a basting brush.

4. Place one large spoonful of batter in the center of the waffle iron and close the lid. Apply pressure for 10 seconds and then cook as per the instructions for your waffle iron. Use a fork to help remove the cooked waffle.

5. Repeat with a little more coconut oil and another large spoonful of batter until all the batter is used up. Makes 12 to 14 whole waffles.

6. Once the waffles are cool, place them in large Ziploc bags and store in the freezer. To defrost, break apart a waffle, place in the microwave for 20 seconds, and then pop it in the toaster on the lowest setting. It's a quick and easy snack, breakfast, or post-workout meal.

## QUINOA
# PORRIDGE

Quinoa has become quite popular over the past several years. This ancient food comes from the Andean region of South America and is loaded with anti-inflammatory phytonutrients. This nutrient-rich food is actually a seed, not a grain, and belongs to the same botanical family as spinach and beets. Make sure to rinse your quinoa before cooking. If you're opposed to quinoa, you could substitute steel cut oats or another complex carbohydrate.

**PREP TIME: 5 MINUTES**
**COOK TIME: 15 MINUTES**
**SERVINGS: 3**

| | |
|---|---|
| 1 | cup quinoa |
| 2 | cups unsweetened almond milk |
| 1 | tablespoon maple syrup |
| $\frac{1}{2}$ | vanilla bean or $\frac{1}{2}$ teaspoon vanilla extract |
| 1 | tablespoon almond butter |
| $\frac{1}{4}$ | cup chopped almonds |

1. In a small saucepan, add the quinoa and almond milk. Cook over high heat until not quite boiling; reduce the mixture to a simmer.

2. Add in the maple syrup, vanilla bean or extract, and almond butter. Cover, reduce the heat to low, and cook for 15 minutes, stirring occasionally. If the mixture appears too thick, add more almond milk or water as necessary.

3. Serve with the chopped almonds on top. Leftover porridge keeps well in the fridge for a week.

## QUINOA
# PANCAKES

We use these quinoa pancakes as a quick, healthy snack before training. They can be high in calories, so don't make them too big. Like the waffles, they freeze well, so you can make a batch that will last a few weeks. They are also handy to pack in a sandwich bag as a snack if you are out for the day. This makes 6 to 8 hand-size pancakes and will keep in the fridge for a week. To reheat, place in a toaster or microwave.

**PREP TIME: 7 MINUTES**
**COOK TIME: 30 MINUTES**
**SERVINGS: 8**

2 tablespoons flaxseed or 2 eggs

2 cups spelt flour

$\frac{1}{2}$ cup almond meal

$\frac{1}{4}$ cup chia seeds

$\frac{1}{2}$ cup rolled oats

1 cup cooked quinoa

1 vanilla bean or 1 teaspoon vanilla extract

$\frac{1}{2}$ teaspoon baking powder

$\frac{1}{2}$ teaspoon baking soda

1 liter unsweetened almond milk

Coconut oil

Maple syrup

1. Option 1: Flaxseed can replace eggs in this recipe. Start by grinding them in a coffee grinder. In a small dish, mix the flaxseed meal with 4 tablespoons water. Stir until you have an egg-like consistency, adding a little more water if necessary. Set aside.

   Option 2: Beat 2 eggs with a small amount of water or almond milk.

2. In a large bowl, place the flour, almond meal, chia seeds, rolled oats, quinoa, vanilla, baking powder, and baking soda.

3. Add half the almond milk, then add either the flax egg or beaten eggs. Stir and add the remaining almond milk. If the batter is too thick, add more almond milk as necessary.

4. In a large skillet, heat 1 teaspoon of coconut oil over medium heat.

5. When the skillet is hot, place a large spoonful of batter in the pan. You can make 2 or 3 pancakes at once, depending on the size you choose. Once the first side is cooked, flip over and cook on the other side.

6. Serve the pancakes with a teaspoon of maple syrup.

# TABBOULEH CHICKPEA
# SALAD

Anytime you open a can of beans, you're off to a good start. This is another perfect Four-Pack dish that is easy to prepare and keeps well in the refrigerator for several days.

**PREP TIME: 15 MINUTES**
**COOK TIME: 2 MINUTES**
**SERVINGS: 3**

| | |
|---|---|
| 2 | bunches parsley, curly or flat leaf |
| 1 | large tomato or 1 handful baby tomatoes |
| 1/2 | white onion, diced |
| 3 | spring onions, chopped |
| 2 | cloves garlic, minced |
| 1 | teaspoon ghee, olive oil, or butter |
| 1 | can (15 ounces) garbanzo beans (chickpeas), drained and rinsed |
| | Salt and pepper |
| | Juice of 1 lemon |

1. Wash, pat dry, and chop the parsley. Place in a large mixing bowl.

2. Dice the large tomato or cut the baby tomatoes in half. Add to the bowl with the onions and garlic.

3. In a large saucepan over medium heat, add the ghee and garbanzos with a sprinkle of salt and pepper to taste. Toss for a few minutes and set aside.

4. Once the garbanzos are cool, add them to the bowl with the other ingredients.

5. Squeeze lemon juice over the ingredients and toss until well combined. This salad stores well in the fridge for a week.

# SPINACH AND
# BEANS

It doesn't get any easier than spinach and beans. If you can open a can of beans, heat them up in a pan, and add several handfuls of spinach, you're there! If you don't feel like using fresh garlic, powder will do. Or just add a little salt and pepper. Add two eggs to this dish and you will have an inexpensive, healthy meal in no time.

**PREP TIME: 5 MINUTES**
**COOK TIME: 3 MINUTES**
**SERVINGS: 3**

| | |
|---|---|
| 1 | tablespoon extra virgin olive oil |
| 4 | cloves garlic, minced |
| 2 | cans (15 ounces) great northern beans or garbanzo beans, drained and rinsed |
| 1 | teaspoon tomato paste |
| 1 | teaspoon agave |
| | Salt and cracked black pepper |
| 5 | cups spinach leaves |

1. In a large skillet, heat the olive oil over medium-low heat. Add the garlic and cook until soft, stirring often. Add the beans to the skillet and stir.

2. Increase the heat to medium and add the tomato paste, agave, a little salt, and some pepper.

3. As soon as the beans are heated through (only a few minutes), turn off the heat and add the spinach until slightly wilted.

## BANZA PASTA WITH ROASTED
# CHERRY TOMATOES

Banza is a new company that set out to create a pasta using garbanzo beans, and they succeeded. Their pasta holds sauce well and has a good texture. A serving of Banza pasta has 25 grams of protein and 13 grams of fiber, compared to regular pasta's 7 grams of protein and 3 grams of fiber. Hard to beat those numbers. If you are ready to reduce the amount of grains in your diet and would still like to eat pasta, give this a try.

**PREP TIME: 5 MINUTES**
**COOK TIME: 20 MINUTES**
**SERVINGS: 2**

1 small container (8 ounces) cherry tomatoes

1 tablespoon extra virgin olive oil

Cracked black pepper

1 liter water

1 cup Banza pasta

1 teaspoon grated Parmesan cheese

1. Preheat the oven to 350°F. Line a small baking pan with parchment paper.

2. Rinse the cherry tomatoes in some water and place them in the prepared pan. Drizzle them with the olive oil and sprinkle with some pepper.

3. Place in the oven for 15 minutes.

4. Meanwhile, in a medium saucepan, bring the water to a boil.

5. Add the pasta, return to a boil, and then reduce the heat to medium so the pasta has rolling movement. Cook the pasta as directed on the package.

6. Remove the tomatoes from the oven and shake the pan to ensure the tomatoes don't stick. Place them back in the oven for another 5 minutes.

7. Drain the pasta and serve with the roasted cherry tomatoes, grated Parmesan, and extra pepper.

# SOUPS

## BROCCOLI AND ALMOND
# SOUP

PREP TIME: 15 MINUTES
COOK TIME: 25 MINUTES
SERVINGS: 5

If you are just starting out and are looking for something new to eat, look no further. This is a very simple soup to make, and it's hard to believe there is no cream in the recipe. This is Ryan's favorite soup and is as healthy as it gets. Make the effort and give it a try.

1 large head broccoli, washed and cut into small florets

1 large white onion, diced

1 liter unsweetened almond milk

1 tablespoon extra virgin olive oil

2 tablespoons almond butter

1 tablespoon apple cider vinegar

Salt and cracked black pepper

1 teaspoon toasted almond flakes

1. In a medium saucepan, add the broccoli, onion, and almond milk and cook over medium to high heat until almost boiling. Reduce the heat to a simmer and cook for 15-20 minutes until the onion and broccoli are soft.

2. Allow the mixture to cool. Pour into a blender.

3. Add the olive oil and almond butter and blend on high for 30 seconds.

4. With the blender on the lowest setting, add the apple cider vinegar. Blend for another 15 seconds on low.

5. Season the soup with salt and pepper and garnish with toasted flaked almonds.

# LENTIL
# SOUP

Lentils, a member of the legume family, rank high on the Four-Pack superfood list. Lentils are high in fiber, folic acid, and potassium and support heart health while reducing LDL cholesterol. This soup freezes well or can last for 10 days in the fridge. It's also high in protein and fiber.

**PREP TIME: 15 MINUTES**
**COOK TIME: 90 MINUTES**
**SERVINGS: 14**

| | |
|---|---|
| 1 | tablespoon extra virgin olive oil |
| 1 | brown onion, diced |
| 2 | stalks celery, chopped |
| 4 | cloves garlic, minced |
| 3 | carrots, chopped |
| 1 | bouillon cube vegetable or chicken stock |
| 4 | cups green lentils |
| 3 | cups red lentils |
| 1 | can unsalted diced tomatoes |
| 1 | bay leaf |
| | Salt and cracked black pepper |

1. In a large pot, heat the olive oil over medium-low heat. Add the onion with a drizzle of water, cover, and let sweat for a few minutes.

2. Add the celery, garlic, and carrots and cook over low heat until soft.

3. Add the stock cube, green lentils, red lentils, tomatoes, bay leaf, and enough water to just cover all the ingredients. Bring to a boil and then reduce to a simmer.

4. Cook for 90 minutes, stirring every 30 minutes.

5. Add salt and pepper to taste before serving.

# BLACK BEAN
# SOUP

It's hard to find a better food than legumes to add to your diet. High in fiber, inexpensive, and low in sugar, beans stabilize blood sugar and promote satiety. They're also as easy as any food to prepare. The most common way they are packaged is in cans, and there is nothing wrong with eating them this way. Once prepared, this black bean soup provides a quick, easy, and delicious meal that can be combined with any type of protein or leafy vegetable, ticking all the boxes for an ideal Four-Pack meal. This soup will last for a week in the fridge. You can also freeze single servings.

**PREP TIME: 5 MINUTES**
**COOK TIME: 4 TO 6 HOURS**
**SERVINGS: 5**

| | |
|---|---|
| 2 | (15 ounces) cans black beans |
| 6 | cups vegetable broth |
| 1 | yellow onion, diced |
| 3 | cloves garlic, minced |
| 1 | teaspoon chili powder |
| 1 | teaspoon cumin |
| $1/2$ | teaspoon oregano |
| 1 | avocado, sliced |

1. In a large saucepan or slow cooker, add the black beans, vegetable broth, onion, garlic, chili powder, cumin, and oregano.

2. If using a saucepan, bring to a boil and then reduce to a simmer. If using a slow cooker, cook on high for 1 hour and then reduce to low. Stir occasionally.

3. Cook for 4 to 6 hours. The broth will reduce over time, but add a little water throughout the cooking process if it appears too thick.

4. Serve with slices of avocado on top.

# QUICK WHITE AND BLACK BEAN
# CHILI SOUP

A healthy bean soup doesn't have to take the afternoon to prepare. Canned beans are convenient, and a pot of delicious, healthy bean soup is not far away. A bowl with leftover chicken and veggies is another quick Four-Pack meal that's ready in no time.

**PREP TIME: 10 MINUTES**
**COOK TIME: 25 MINUTES**
**SERVINGS: 4**

| | |
|---|---|
| 1 | teaspoon extra virgin olive oil |
| ½ | medium onion, chopped |
| 4 | cloves garlic, minced |
| 1 | whole green or red bell pepper, chopped |
| ½ | red bell pepper, chopped |
| 1 | teaspoon cumin |
| 1 | teaspoon oregano |
| ½ | teaspoon chili powder |
| ½ | teaspoon cayenne pepper |
| ¼ | teaspoon black pepper |
| 1 | teaspoon lime juice |
| 3 | tablespoons tomato paste |
| 2 | large tomatoes, chopped into small pieces |
| ¾ | teaspoon salt |
| 1 | can (15 ounces) organic great northern white beans, drained and rinsed |
| 1 | can (15 ounces) organic black beans, drained and rinsed |
| 1 | bouillon cube vegetable or chicken stock |
| 2 | cups water |
| | A few sprigs cilantro, chopped |
| 1 | avocado, sliced |

1. In a large saucepan, heat the olive oil over medium heat. Add the onion, garlic, and a drizzle of water and cook, stirring occasionally, about 5 minutes.

2. Add the bell pepper, cumin, oregano, chili powder, cayenne pepper, and black pepper and cook, stirring, for 3 minutes.

3. Add the lime juice, tomato paste, tomatoes, and salt and stir. Then add the beans, bouillon cube, and water. Cover the pot and cook for 15 minutes.

4. Serve with the cilantro, avocado slices, and an additional sprinkle of black pepper.

# PROTEIN

The benefits that protein provides for weight loss are well established. Now turn your focus to where these foods come from: The process by which most of the fish, chicken, eggs, and fish you eat are raised usually leaves a lot to be desired. Only consume free-range or wild organic protein–it may cost a little more, but the investment is worth it.

# OMELET

**PREP TIME: 5 MINUTES**
**COOK TIME: 3 MINUTES**
**SERVINGS: 1**

Eggs are among the most nutritious foods on the planet, high in protein, B vitamins, and choline. But all not all eggs are created equal. Hens raised on pasture and/or fed omega-3-enriched feeds will create eggs containing better quality fats. They are the perfect food for when you travel, found in every breakfast restaurant or room service menu. Learn to cook eggs three ways—as an omelet, poached, and fried—and you'll be able to create a low-cost, great-tasting, and healthy meal whenever you'd like.

| | |
|---|---|
| 1 | teaspoon extra virgin olive oil |
| 1/4 | small yellow onion, finely chopped |
| 1 | plum tomato, finely chopped (about 1/3 cup) |
| | Handful spinach (fresh or frozen) |
| 5 | egg whites or 3 whole eggs |
| 1 | tablespoon water |
| | Salt and freshly ground black pepper |

1. In a large skillet, heat the olive oil over medium heat. Add the onion and a pinch of salt and sauté until soft.

2. Add the tomatoes and cook for 1 minute, stirring. Add in the spinach and cook until it begins to wilt.

3. Remove the skillet from the heat; cover and keep warm.

4. In a separate bowl, whisk together the egg whites, water, and a pinch of salt until frothy. Add to a separate, lightly oiled skillet and cook over medium heat for 1½ to 2 minutes. Occasionally, use a spatula to lift up the eggs and allow the runny egg to flow underneath.

5. Spoon the spinach mixture onto half the omelet, fold over, and slide onto a plate. Add salt and pepper to taste.

# ROAST CHICKEN

This classic works well with leftovers or straight out of the oven. Spend a little more for organic, free-range chicken. Bake a large batch twice a week and you'll have a quick, healthy meal available in less than 5 minutes.

**COOK TIME: 30 MINUTES**
**PREP TIME: 3 MINUTES**
**SERVINGS: 3**

3-5 pounds chicken pieces, legs, thighs, and/or breasts (bone in and skin on if using breasts)

1-2 tablespoons extra virgin olive oil

1 teaspoon salt

½ teaspoon black pepper

1. Preheat the oven to 400°F.

2. Rinse the chicken pieces and pat dry with paper towels. Transfer to a mixing bowl.

3. Toss the chicken with 1 tablespoon of the olive oil, salt, and pepper. Add more olive oil as needed to coat each piece. Sprinkle with additional salt and pepper until the pieces are evenly seasoned.

4. Transfer the seasoned chicken pieces to a baking sheet and arrange them skin-side up in a single layer, leaving a bit of space between each piece.

5. Bake for 20 to 30 minutes or until the chicken is opaque throughout and the meat registers at least 165°F in the thickest part.

# GRILLED SALMON

Wild salmon is listed on every superfood list, and with good reason: The combination of healthy protein and essential fats is hard to beat.

**PREP TIME: 5 MINUTES**
**COOK TIME: 7 MINUTES**
**SERVINGS: 4**

1½ pounds wild salmon

**MARINADE**

3 cloves garlic, minced

3 tablespoons olive oil

2 tablespoons lemon juice

1 teaspoon salt

1 teaspoon black pepper

1. Place the salmon in a resealable plastic bag.

2. In a small bowl, whisk together the garlic, olive oil, lemon juice, salt, and pepper. Pour into the bag with the salmon and place in the refrigerator to marinate for 1 hour.

3. Place the fillets over a medium-hot grill or grill pan. Cook for 3 to 4 minutes on each side.

# TUNA
# SALAD

Tuna is all protein, easy to find, and relatively inexpensive. Yes, there are some concerns about mercury levels with fish, especially predatory fish such as tuna. That said, for many it is an affordable source of protein that is quick to prepare. If you are in a rush and need to modify this recipe, just adding avocado and a little salt and pepper makes a great meal.

**PREP TIME: 7 MINUTES**
**SERVINGS: 1**

1 can (5 ounces) unsalted albacore tuna in water, drained

1 stalk celery, chopped into small pieces

6 sprigs parsley or coriander, leaves chopped

1 clove garlic, minced

½ avocado, mashed

 Juice from ½ lime

1 tablespoon hempseed

 Salt and cracked black pepper

1. Place the tuna in a small mixing bowl. Add the celery, parsley, garlic, mashed avocado, lime juice, and hempseed and mix together well.

2. Taste before seasoning with salt and pepper. This is even better than regular tuna salad!


# BAKED
# HALIBUT

If you are new to fish, it's hard to go wrong with halibut. This mild white fish is caught in the cold waters of the north Pacific Ocean and is easy to bake, grill, or pan-fry.

**PREP TIME: 5 MINUTES**
**COOK TIME: 12 MINUTES**
**SERVINGS: 2**

1 pound halibut, 1 large fillet or several smaller ones

1 teaspoon olive oil

2 cloves garlic

1 teaspoon lemon zest

2 tablespoons lemon juice

4 sprigs fresh parsley

 Salt and black pepper

1. Preheat the oven to 400°F.

2. In a large nonstick baking dish, add the halibut skin-side down and drizzle with the olive oil.

3. Top each fillet with the garlic, lemon zest, lemon juice, and parsley, dividing evenly. Season with salt and pepper.

4. Bake for 12 to 15 minutes, until the halibut flakes easily when tested with a fork.

# SALAD DRESSINGS, SAUCES, AND DIPS

## HONEY MUSTARD

Most commercial salad dressings are loaded with unhealthy ingredients, especially low-quality oils. Having a few different versions ready in the refrigerator can make eating your veggies easier.

**PREP TIME: 5 TO 7 MINUTES**
**SERVINGS: 2**

1 tablespoon honey

2 tablespoons Dijon mustard

1 clove garlic

Juice of 1 lemon

1 tablespoon apple cider vinegar

1/2 cup nutritional yeast

Cracked black pepper

1. In a blender, add the honey, mustard, garlic, lemon juice, apple cider vinegar, nutritional yeast, and a pinch of pepper and blend together for 10 seconds. If making by hand, mix together the honey and mustard first; mince the garlic and add with the lemon juice, apple cider vinegar, nutritional yeast, and black pepper.

## OLIVE OIL AND LEMON

If you need a quick salad dressing, look no further. This recipe swaps out the traditional vinegar with lemon for a light, healthy dressing.

**PREP TIME: 2 MINUTES**
**SERVINGS: 1**

1 tablespoon extra virgin olive oil

Juice of 1 lemon

Salt and cracked black pepper

1. In a small bowl, whisk together the olive oil and lemon juice. Season to taste with salt and pepper.

# PEANUT
# SAUCE

This recipe is a healthy version of the peanut sauce served at Thai restaurants. It's quick and easy to make and is a delicious addition to many dishes.

**PREP TIME: 3 MINUTES**
**SERVINGS: 1**

| | |
|---|---|
| 1 | tablespoon unsalted creamy peanut butter |
| 1 | tablespoon apple cider vinegar |
| 1 | tablespoon water |
| ¼ | teaspoon agave |
| 1 | teaspoon low-sodium soy sauce |

1. In a small bowl, whisk together the peanut butter and apple cider vinegar. Once a thick paste forms, mix in the water.

2. Add the agave and soy sauce and mix until well combined. If a thinner peanut sauce is desired, add more water until the desired consistency is achieved.


# PISTACHIO
# PESTO

Pesto is a classic sauce from northern Italy that is traditionally used with pasta. It works great with Banza pasta and also with eggs, meats, or vegetables. Use fresh or freeze for future use.

**PREP TIME: 7 MINUTES**
**FREEZE TIME: 4 HOURS**
**SERVINGS: 12**

| | |
|---|---|
| 1 | cup unsalted pistachios, shelled |
| 1 | tablespoon extra virgin olive oil |
| ½ | cup roughly chopped parsley leaves |
| 1½ | cups packed fresh basil leaves |
| 2 | tablespoons nutritional yeast |
| ¼ | cup water |

1. In a high-powered blender or food processor, add the pistachios, olive oil, parsley, basil, nutritional yeast, and water and blend for 40 seconds.

2. Scrape out or spoon mixture into an ice cube tray. Place in the freezer for at least 4 hours.

3. Once the pesto is frozen, remove the ice cube tray from the freezer and pop out the pesto cubes. Store the cubes in a freezer bag in the freezer.

4. To thaw, in a small saucepan, place 1 to 2 pesto cubes and 1 teaspoon water. Heat over medium-low heat until the cubes are soft enough to break up and stir back into a sauce. The pesto is then ready to serve on pasta or zucchini slaw. Delicious!

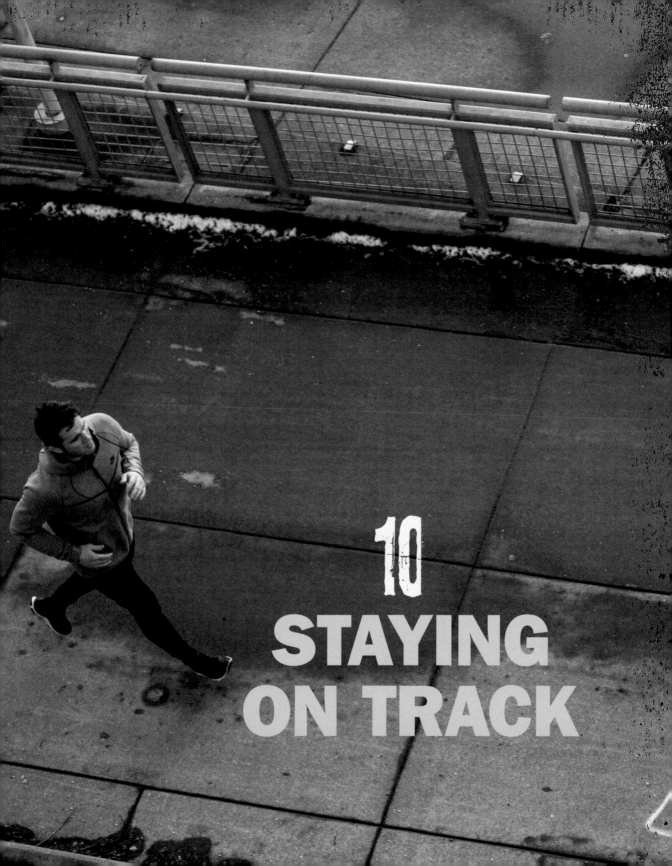

# 10
# STAYING
# ON TRACK

THE DIRTIEST WORD IN THE DIET INDUSTRY IS "TIME." FOR THE SAME REASONS get-rich-quick schemes are so appealing, rapid-weight-loss diets turn us into a bunch of suckers. Who doesn't want to wake up in amazing shape 10 days after starting a new diet and workout regime? The billion-dollar diet industry was built on the back of this all too common human desire—expecting something for nothing. But as you reflect on your life, notice that your biggest accomplishments took time. You don't remember, but it took around a year to learn to walk and several years to avoid going to the bathroom in your pants. If you are a former athlete or a musician, think about how many hours you spent practicing your craft. Not one diet expert wants to tell you: "If you're going to do this right, it's going to take some time." We readily admit this is not as appealing as "Six-Pack Abs in 21 Days!" but like it or not, it's the truth. You didn't gain all that weight overnight, and replacing those behaviors that created the problem is a process. But you were given a powerful tool for this transformation—your brain. And it's masterfully designed to adapt to change at any age.

## PATIENCE VS. PROGRESS

Unless you have a fight to weigh in for, rushing weight loss is almost always a bad idea. The challenge is to balance patience with progress. We've advised lowering your expectations, but this does not mean throwing accountability out the window. Pay attention to the number on your bathroom scale, follow the Four-Pack nutritional guidelines, and push yourself during exercise to elevate your heart rate and build muscle. Patience reduces the anxiety associated with expecting change to happen immediately. Adapt your daily routines to these fundamentals and success is virtually guaranteed. Your System Reset meals have physiological benefits, but they're also a reminder that life is to be lived and enjoyed. Keep it playful and fun and you will get there.

## PROGRESS VS. RESULTS

We love results. We dream about them and work hard to make them a reality. Since you are reading this book, our assumption is that you would like to lose weight. But what happens when you do? Let's say a few months from now you post a picture of your awesome new four-pack. Then what? "Then what" is where so many people fall off. Talk to anyone who has achieved a significant life accomplishment and they'll tell you: After the initial rush of excitement and celebration wears off, "then what" hits them like a brick to the head. This has to be where the whole concept of living in the moment comes from. Some ultra-successful individual achieved all his dreams, only to realize those accomplishments didn't bring the fulfillment that was promised. It turns out the process is the reward. Keeping the majority of your focus on progress, and less on the end goal, creates success that lasts for decades.

## PROCRASTINATION

Confession: We procrastinated writing this section on procrastination. It lasted only two days, but the struggle was real—so you're not alone when it comes to putting things off. In this case, it was not that big of a deal, but many people turn procrastination into a full-time hobby. It's difficult to find an area in life where procrastination is more prevalent than losing weight. It's one of the reasons crash diets and weight-loss gimmicks are so popular. We put off healthy eating and exercise until one day we can't stand it anymore. Then there's a mad rush to lose as much weight as quickly as possible. This is a terrible way to approach the challenge and is one reason why 85 percent of people who diet this year will gain all the weight back plus a little extra for good measure. But what if you never procrastinated again for the rest of your life? Imagine what you would accomplish?

Our competitive nature would like us to write a simple explanation for understanding procrastination, but unfortunately, like the world's obesity problem, there are several contributing factors that muddy the waters. Neuroscientists may not have pinpointed the exact source of the problem, but from what we do know there are at least two parts of the brain involved. The first is your limbic system, which is the instinctual part of your brain, highly involved with emotions and the fight-or-flight response. Its function is to act quickly to keep you alive. But as you know, emotions are often irrational and if not kept in check lead to poor decision-making. The second area is the slower-acting prefrontal cortex, which is responsible for setting goals and storing dreams for the future.

Researchers at Case Western Reserve University published a study on procrastination in *Psychological Science* in 1997. It turns out students who procrastinated scored lower grades than non-procrastinators and reported high levels of stress and illness. Although their work may have been turned in on time, it just wasn't as good as it could have been.

Taking the time to consider where you would like your life to be in 12 months gives you a target to aim for. But learning to take action the moment procrastination creeps in is the key to long-term results.

Let's put this into a real-world scenario. Let's say it's time to do your taxes. The due date is coming up, and the box of receipts in your closet needs sorting. Your limbic system does not care about penalties from the IRS. The future does not exist in that part of your brain, and getting rid of those uncomfortable emotions is its top priority. The "flight" reaction in your fight-or-flight response is much easier, especially when your opponent is paperwork or a stack of dirty dishes in the sink. These small, daily events don't put up much of a fight when they are ignored, but down the road the consequences can be severe. The prefrontal cortex is much better than the limbic system at carefully considering all aspects of a challenge, but this ability comes with a price. This rational part of the brain is slower to respond than the more instinctual limbic system. Taxes can wait. Someone else will wash those dishes. Let's see what's happening on YouTube/chaelsonnen.

In the most practical sense, overcoming procrastination requires you to become a better decision maker. If your brain is capable of making 38 thousand trillion calculations a second, surely it can figure out a way to get your to-do list completed. Whatever parts of your brain are involved with decision-making, they become stronger with use. If you're the type who overthinks and needs to ask 10 different people their opinions before making up your mind, practice making decisive, small decisions every day for 2 weeks. You'll have many opportunities. The next time you are out to dinner in a restaurant, give yourself 30 seconds to scan the menu and pick something. Then forget about it and eat whatever the waiter delivers. Keep your emotions in check throughout the whole meal.

The simplest approach to overcoming procrastination is to train your brain to act the moment indecisiveness arises. You know exactly what the initial sensation of procrastination feels like. Start small: When you see a dish in the sink, instead of walking by, stop,

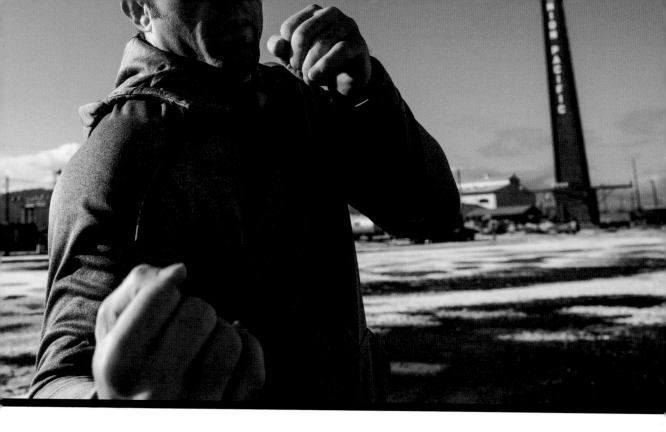

wash it, and put it away. Procrastination is a habit that has been conditioned over years of wanting to avoid uncomfortable emotions. Action breaks this pattern and sets you on a new path.

One more thing: Don't expect procrastination to disappear. It's not an infectious disease that can be eradicated with a new medication. It's natural to want to avoid tasks you don't enjoy, especially when a more engaging alternative is close by. But the amount of power that procrastination has over you is entirely your decision. Just as you can expect to get hungry several times a day, you can also count on the urge to procrastinate to appear daily as well. But just as hunger is not a bad thing, neither is the sensation of procrastination. They are both reminders of an immediate opportunity to make a decision that will move you closer to your long-term weight-loss goals. At the end of the day, procrastination is not something that can be eliminated—just like hunger, it needs to be managed.

## ACTIVATION ENERGY

It takes a certain amount of oomph, or activation energy, when starting anything new. Without activation energy it's easy to fall into the trap of "starting tomorrow." Why not? You can feel comfortable in the next 30 seconds by consuming a cheeseburger. In the short term, starting tomorrow doesn't mean much; it's only one day. But those days sure do add up. How many Mondays have passed in your life where you were supposed to start something new? And each time you give in and postpone your start, you become a little weaker. Over the long term, the impact of those decisions can be catastrophic.

Activation energy is not something you generate once and that's it–you'll need to refresh it daily. But it's easier to create when you're doing things you enjoy. This is one reason why having compelling goals and an inspiring vision for your future is so important. Make this work for you by finding healthy foods you enjoy eating. Create workouts that are fun and find friends to join you. Try something new or something old; be creative, this is how you succeed.

Incentives play a significant role in the amount of internal drive you are able to muster. Often the best incentives come with a deadline attached. It works for fighters, authors writing a book, and you. Signing with the UFC provides a strong incentive that makes getting up and going to the gym easier. A bride-to-be also knows the power of a deadline. Fitting into that dress on her wedding day provides a powerful incentive to look her best. So create incentives that inspire you to make a move.

## PAY ATTENTION

Chances are you're making some silly mistakes, like adding extra sugar in your coffee or drinking excess calories when water would do. Are you ignoring opportunities to be active? Ten pushups and a walk around the block after dinner take very little effort. Could you be stretching on the floor while watching TV at night instead of lying on the couch? Becoming more active has a powerful impact on how you feel throughout the day and night. Each little opportunity you find builds momentum and anchors new habits.

Here are a few suggestions.

- For the next few days, look at the calorie count and grams of sugar of everything you drink. Drink whatever you'd like, just be aware of what's in the bottle.

- Daily exercise challenge:
  - 10, 50, 10, 250, 500, or 1,000 pushups in a day
  - 100 air squats after each meal
  - Lunges between two street light poles
  - Planks: 30 seconds, or 1 to 5 minutes
  - 100 jumping jacks
- Turn off any screens an hour before bed.
- Wake up 30 minutes earlier than usual.
- Buy a new water bottle and carry it throughout the day.

## LOWER YOUR EXPECTATIONS

We're all for dreaming big and working hard to achieve lofty goals, but there's a time and a place for low expectations—and this is one of those times. If you have any apprehension or doubt, start slow. Really slow. Whatever is just above "zero effort," that's the place. Here's an example: Drink one less soda today. That's it, nothing else. Leave one bite of food on your plate at the end of a meal and do three pushups. Big goals are not always the answer. Consistent action—even small efforts—pays dividends and keeps expectations in check. The best tennis players in the world play the point, not the game. If you're aiming to lose 30 pounds, you have to get to 29 first.

## LIVING IS GOOD, SABOTAGE IS NOT

There will come a time when it's been 2 weeks since you've worked out and the scale reads 6 pounds heavier than you'd like. Maybe that four-pack has morphed into a two-pack. What you do in these moments is more important than any diet or workout program. You've got two choices the next time you are hungry: eat something healthy, or sabotage everything because you're a little frustrated.

### If You Fail, Here's Why

Who are we kidding? There is no if, just when. Screw-ups will happen for the rest of your life, and since we've established that failure is part of the process, let's all agree to have a little forgiveness in our hearts, learn from our mistakes, and move on. Successful people fail a lot, but they don't see missteps as the end of the road, just a learning experience or an opportunity for reassessment. When you drift off course, it's typically because of one of the following reasons.

- **You were not prepared.** Life will catch you off guard. Remember, your body can only think short term. For example, when you get hungry, you'll instinctively look for a way to fix that. Most of us have a few bad eating habits that are easy to revert to, but preparation will steer you away from these temptations. Tupperware is your friend, and it takes only a little more effort to prepare eight pieces of chicken than it does one. Leftovers can be transformed into a healthy meal in minutes.

- **You're stressed out.** Food is a powerful way to change your emotional state. You can try to fight it, but this response is hardwired into the brain. When we eat, powerful pain-relieving chemicals similar to heroin are released in the brain. Scientists call it ingestion analgesia, or pain relief delivered through eating. Thankfully, you are not limited to food as your only choice to relieve stress—exercise, breathing, prayer, music, connecting with friends . . . there are many more options. Pick a few and put them to work.

- **You're seeing yourself as a victim.** This is a nicer way of saying, "Quit being a . . . ." Victims feel as though they lack control over what happens to them, including their emotions. Making excuses for what's wrong in your life reinforces this victim mentality. You will only move forward by looking at your problems from a different perspective. It can't happen any other way. We have all made mistakes before, so when they happen, don't burn the house down. Just because things don't go your way doesn't mean life is over. Take a deep breath, reassess, and have a protein shake.

## Red Flags

Red flags are warning signs that you're veering off course. Even if you miss them, it doesn't mean they're not there. We are constantly given feedback from our body to let us know how our lifestyle is serving us. Learn to spot these red flags and you'll save yourself unnecessary pain and frustration. Here are a few to watch out for.

- **Dark urine:** If you go to the bathroom and your pee is yellow, you're dehydrated. It's common to mistake thirst for hunger, and we often eat when we should be drinking water. Get into the habit of carrying a water bottle around with you. It makes staying hydrated easier and helps cut down on the amount of calories you consume each day.

- **Skipping breakfast:** Some people are just not hungry in the morning and that's okay, but be sure there's protein and fiber in your first meal of the day to help stabilize blood sugar. If you are rushed in the morning, have some go-to food like a protein smoothie that you can grab on your way out the door.

- **Staring at the refrigerator:** Nothing happened inside the refrigerator since the last time you checked. Boredom and a restless mind frequently lead to snacking, and these unplanned calories add up. Eat on a schedule so you know when you're actually hungry and need to eat, and you're not just snacking because you're bored or feeling stressed.

- **Waking up groggy:** Poor quality sleep can lead to significant health issues. Establish a bedtime schedule and minimize TV and computer time in the hour or two before going to sleep. Learn to unwind at the end of the day without technology so you can properly rest, recover, and be ready to tackle tomorrow with energy.

- **Weighing yourself multiple times a day:** This is a common beginner mistake. Expectations are high, and there's a certain amount of stress that occurs with change. This is why we emphasize taking your time, because losing weight quickly often leads to a rebound effect. Finding ways to remain calm and patient during the process is important for long-term success, so restrict yourself to checking the scale once a day at most. Better yet, once or twice a week, to relieve yourself of that daily (or hourly) pressure.

- **Eating late:** Late-night eating is often linked to anxiety and stress and is not real hunger. But if you think you are truly hungry, then have a small snack like a handful of nuts or a bowl of blueberries to make going to bed easier. We use kombucha tea while cutting weight. It is the best thing we've found to cut hunger late at night.

## Tips for Staying on Track While Eating Out

Cooking at home is one thing, but dining out can be challenging when trying to eat a healthy meal. Thankfully, this is an easy one to navigate. Here are a few tips to help you stick to your goals without having to give up your social life. Experiment the next time you go out to eat.

- **Read the menu before you go.** If you're not familiar with the menu, read it beforehand. You'll be more social at the table, and making a quick decision about your meal makes you look confident. The chances of you ordering the fettuccine alfredo increase when you're hungry, distracted, or feeling like everyone is looking at you. Plan ahead. This only takes a few minutes and helps avoid snap decisions you'll regret on the drive home.

- **Don't arrive hungry.** If you sit down at the table famished, your chances of overeating increase dramatically. Eating a high-protein snack such as Greek yogurt ahead of time will help take the edge off your hunger.

- **Question your food.** The way food is prepared greatly influences calorie content. If the menu is not clear, ask your server how the dish is prepared and request a different method of cooking such as grilling, steaming, or with light oil if necessary. Most servers are used to these sorts of questions.

- **Enjoy your company.** Going out to eat isn't just about food—you're there to connect. Paying attention to the people you're eating with will help you eat slower. Not only will you strengthen relationships, you'll also enjoy the experience more and your body will be thankful.

- **Skip the buffet.** It's a buffet! Which means it's socially acceptable to eat three plates of food, right? Most of us have difficulty estimating portion size to begin with, but the allure of eating as much as you want without having to pay more drives many people to "get their money's worth." If you do end up at a buffet, eat a large salad first, and then use a smaller plate for the rest of your meal. If you must, have one dessert instead of six.

- **Avoid soft drinks and lemonade.** Every restaurant offers water, so feel free to drink it. Soft drinks and lemonade are loaded with sugar—the exact type of calories you want to avoid. If you must drink something with flavor, ask for unsweetened iced tea.

- **Get your dressings on the side.** Restaurant salads are usually loaded with dressing. Order it on the side so you can have a better idea of how much you're eating, or better yet, request olive oil and balsamic vinegar so you can control the ratio and amount of each ingredient yourself.

- **Order off-menu.** Many chefs are happy to adjust a recipe to meet your needs. Most meat, chicken, fish, and veggies can be grilled or steamed, which are healthier and lower-calorie methods of cooking. Don't be afraid to ask.

- **Send the bread back.** In the moment, this is a tough decision to make. But warm bread before dinner is a temptation you don't need while you're hungry and waiting for your meal to arrive.

- **Start with a soup and salad.** Beginning with a soup or salad can help reduce the amount of total calories you'll eat during your meal. Just make sure it's a cup of soup, not a bowl, and preferably not full of noodles. Opt for broth-based soups when you can.

- **Keep each meal in perspective.** One meal never ruined anyone's ability to lose weight. Even if you're not scheduled for a System Reset meal and one slips through the cracks, it's not the end of the world. The more weight you lose and the more muscle you build, the easier it will be to deal with an occasional slip-up.

# EPILOGUE

IMAGINE THIS IS THE MOMENT THE CAGE DOOR CLOSES BEHIND YOU. IT'S JUST you and your opponent. To come out on top with your hand raised in victory, you must find a way to win. After reading this book, you now have a better understanding of how to lose weight than the vast majority of people. It's not an easy task, so expect to make mistakes. But when you do, remember you can always find your way back. The real battle you face is the one you wage between your ears. Your success will be determined by how you manage expectations, emotions, and your environment.

You picked up this book for a reason, and while you've been reading, someone in the exact same position as you ate a Big Mac. As you finish your next workout, with your metabolism kicked into high gear, someone else will have crushed another beer while flipping through the channels sitting on the sofa. Who would you bet on? Our money's on you.

Confidence is needed to succeed, and it's built from an accumulation of small victories. Each time you reinforce a new habit, your confidence grows. Each time you put your foot down and refuse to run old, unhealthy patterns from your past, you'll become stronger. When you catch yourself slipping up and immediately right the ship without beating yourself up, you become more capable. This process will be ongoing.

Having a realistic game plan is essential, but it's worthless without the willingness to step up and do the work. No one can do it for you. Every day, find opportunities for small victories and tailor your meals and workouts to fit your personal style so you're in the best position to win. Planning doesn't require much time or effort. Remember, this isn't just a diet or a training program. It's you changing, moving forward and creating a new future for yourself and those you love.

You may have realized over the course of reading this book that some of the expectations you used to have for yourself were not entirely realistic. If that's the case, how good does it feel to shed that excess baggage? Carrying around standards that no one could possibly achieve takes its toll. Now you can really start living. When you are no longer tied to the idea that there's one "right way," it frees up energy to pursue a new approach. You'll tap into resources you didn't know were available while becoming more flexible, patient, and satisfied with life. That's all most of us really want, and it's so much better than any number on a scale.

Remember, the Four-Pack plan is not a magic pill—success requires daily maintenance and refinements. The beauty of this approach is that it allows you to adjust your meals and workouts in a way that supports your biology and personality. It also places you firmly in control of your own destiny with the know-how to create a winning strategy that works for you. Nothing builds confidence like taking back control of your health. You'll hold your head higher and you'll walk with more purpose in your step.

But before we send you off, there is one question we haven't spent much time on: How long will this take? Well, that depends—it's different for everyone. Are you significantly overweight, or are there 10 stubborn pounds you'd like to see disappear? Wherever you're starting, don't rush. Life is long and there's still plenty of time. One pound a week over the course of the next year adds up—losing 50 pounds is a life-changing event that can potentially add years to your time here on Earth. Think about that for a minute.

Will it really take a year to lose 50 pounds? It can be done sooner, but your chances of keeping the weight off for the long haul increase dramatically when you slow down and take your time. Start to find fulfillment in the process instead of obsessing over the perfect number on a scale. The primary advantage of this slow-paced approach is that it takes the pressure off. It also allows you to become accustomed to doing things differently. With time to practice, make mistakes, and learn, you will improve and give yourself an opportunity to truly integrate these habits into your lifestyle. With enough repetition, almost anything can seem like second nature—even exercise and healthy eating.

Share your success story with us at ultimatefourpack.com. We know you're capable. We'll be extra impressed with the four-packs that are still being flexed in the mirror each morning 12 months after they were first achieved. By that time, everything in this book will be second nature for you. Your body will be so strong and efficient that any System Reset meal will be processed with ease. And for those times when your four-pack becomes a two-pack or even a no-pack, take a step back. Ryan survived a parachute malfunction. Chael failed at the highest level of his sport—three times. And these were not significant tests in the grand scheme of life. You have your own battle stories, those moments that develop character. They serve as reminders that no matter what happens, life goes on—but how your life continues depends on what you do next.

# ACKNOWLEDGMENTS

We're fortunate to have an amazing team behind us: Pat Sonnen, John Parsons, Rachel Kiely, Becca Jenkins, Mimi Solaire, Heath Sims, the Great Roy Pittman, Dave Sanvile, Casey Galpin, Simon Milne, Coach P. J. Nestler, Dr. Andy Galpin and the Center for Sport Performance at CSU Fullerton, Daniel Cormier, and Maxine Allen all contributed to this book, and we are forever grateful for their insight, stories, and inspiration.

Special thanks to our agent, Rob Kirkpatrick; editor, Mark Weinstein; designer, Joanna Williams; art director, Amy King; and photographer, Matt Brush, who–along with the entire team at Rodale–worked tirelessly to make this project a reality. We are stronger with them in our corner.

# ABOUT THE AUTHORS

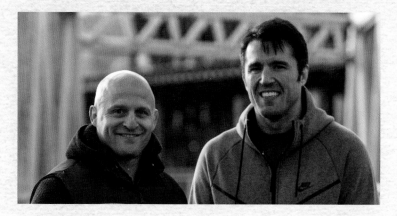

**Chael Sonnen** is a mixed martial arts superstar, volunteer coach, entrepreneur, television commentator, and author. A graduate of the University of Oregon, Sonnen rose to the elite ranks of the Ultimate Fighting Championship. Sonnen's brilliant, incisive, and unique viewpoints have made him a favorite of fans, fellow athletes, and lazy journalists. He was a cast member on *The New Celebrity Apprentice* and also appears regularly as an analyst on ESPN and a commentator for Bellator MMA. Sonnen is the author of one previous book, *The Voice of Reason: A VIP Pass to Enlightenment*. He lives in West Linn, OR.

**Ryan Parsons** is a peak performance expert, veteran MMA coach, manager, and consultant. He received his doctorate in chiropractic medicine from the Southern California University of Health Sciences, Los Angeles College of Chiropractic, after an underwhelming wrestling career. Parsons has worked with world champions in every major fight promotion and is the inventor of Radius Wraps, the first combat sport product to undergo a peer-reviewed university clinical trial. He has cut weight with elite athletes on five continents in all kinds of places—in saunas, steam rooms, hot tubs, hotel rooms, city parks, the beach, and even at an arena under a camera crew's lights. He lives in Los Angeles, CA.

# INDEX

Boldface page references denote photographs. Underscored page references denote boxed text.